Cervical Cancer - Recent Advances and New Perspectives

Edited by Michael Friedrich

Published in London, United Kingdom

Cervical Cancer - Recent Advances and New Perspectives
http://dx.doi.org/10.5772/intechopen.1000389
Edited by Michael Friedrich

Contributors
Natalia Garcia-Becerra, Carlos A. Garcia-Becerra, Leonardo Fernandez-Avila, Jose Roberto Cruz-Lozano, Veronica Soltero-Molinar, Isabel Arias-Gallardo, Sofia Briseida Leyva-Delgado, Angel E. Chávez-Torres, Dalia I. Murillo-Geraldo, Jesús E. Juarez-Garcia, Johanna Melissa Aguayo Joza, Carlos Javier Más López, Guido Enrique Terán Mogro, Luis Santiago Quiroz Fernández, Shirley Elizabeth Pizarro Anchundia, Amy Melissa Loor Aguayo, Joan Manuel Loor Aguayo, Shr, Andha Srivastava, Nara Singh Moirangthem, Arunima Ghosh, Indrajeet Gupta, Madan Lal Brahma Bhatt, Zakariyya Muhammad Bello, Sharafudeen Dahiru Abubakar, Imam Malik Kabir, Lukman Yusuf

First published in London, United Kingdom, 2024 by IntechOpen
IntechOpen is the global imprint of INTECHOPEN LIMITED, registered in England and Wales, registration number: 11086078, 5 Princes Gate Court, London, SW7 2QJ, United Kingdom

British Library Cataloguing-in-Publication Data
A catalogue record for this book is available from the British Library

Additional hard and PDF copies can be obtained from orders@intechopen.com

Cervical Cancer - Recent Advances and New Perspectives
Edited by Michael Friedrich
p. cm.
Print ISBN 978-1-83769-338-2
Online ISBN 978-1-83769-337-5
eBook (PDF) ISBN 978-1-83769-339-9

Meet the editor

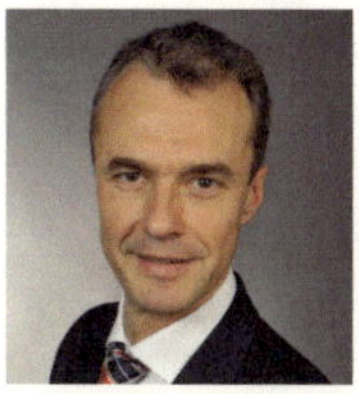

Michael Friedrich is a senior gynecological oncologist and oncological surgeon at Helios Klinikum Krefeld, Germany, and specializes in treating women with breast cancer and gynecological malignancies. He is a certified breast surgeon and has an academic appointment as an associate professor at the University of Schleswig-Holstein, Germany. He has received several awards for his scientific work, which focuses on vitamin D metabolism in gynecologic malignancies and the interaction of DNA-mismatch repair and resistance to chemotherapy. Further research interests are interstitial brachytherapy for recurrences of cervical cancer, the use of innovative therapies in gynecological malignancies, the sentinel lymph node technique in gynecological malignancies, especially in vulvar cancer, and the use of intraoperative intraperitoneal chemotherapy (HIPEC) in ovarian cancer. Dr. Friendrich is a member of several prestigious editorial and scientific boards and a member of Germany's committees for S3-guidelines for cervical, endometrial, vulvar, and breast cancer. He is also a member of the Ethics Committee of the Nordrhein-Westfalen Medical Chamber, the board of directors of the BLFG (Bundesarbeitsgemeinschaft leitender Frauenärzte), the board of the German Society for Gynecology, where he is responsible for developing the continuous medical education curriculum in gynecology, and the Society of Pelvic Surgeons.

Contents

Preface

Cervical cancer is a heterogeneous disease composed of multiple distinct molecular and clinical subtypes. Improvements in the ability to target the underlying drivers of ovarian cancer, combined with advances in surgical techniques, are crucial for developing effective treatments for patients with ovarian cancer. This book addresses recent advances, new perspectives, and applications in the treatment of cervical cancer.

Chapter 1, "Molecular and Cell Biology of Cervical Cancer" by Natalia Garcia-Becerra et al., discusses the molecular and cell biology of cervical cancer in detail, emphasizing the disease's etiology, epidemiology, risk factors, hallmarks, and the main signaling pathways involved. The chapter delves into the characteristics of cancer, such as changes in cell cycle regulation, apoptosis, and cell differentiation, as well as the tumoral microenvironment. It also highlights signal pathways like the PI3K/AKT/mTOR pathway and the Wnt/beta-catenin pathway for their significance in the development of cervical cancer. The chapter thoroughly explains the molecular and cell biology underlying this terrible illness.

Chapter 2, "Radiotherapy in Cervical Cancer" by Shraddha Srivastava et al., examines the important role of radiotherapy in the treatment of cervical cancer. In recent decades, there have been several advancements in radiation therapy treatment techniques. Moving from conventional two-dimensional techniques to advanced techniques like 3D conformal radiation therapy (3D-CRT), intensity-modulated radiation therapy (IMRT), and volumetric-modulated radiation therapy (VMAT) has led to improvement in treatment outcomes. These advanced techniques deliver optimal tumoricidal doses to tumor volumes and minimal doses to the normal tissues around the tumor and can reduce toxicity more effectively than conventional techniques. These external beam radiotherapy (EBRT) techniques, along with brachytherapy, play a significant role in the treatment of gynecological cancer. Compared to point-based dose brachytherapy planning, advanced image-based brachytherapy is associated with better local control and lower toxicity.

Chapter 3, "The Costs of Cervical Cancer Treatment with a Social Focus" by Johanna Melissa Aguayo Joza, focuses on the value creation system in the strategic management of costs associated with diseases, showing the need to focus the analysis on the activities involved in management, since they detail all the interrelated actions to achieve efficiency in treatment, particularly in cervical cancer. The design of the value chain is important in the economic context in which it is created and for the agents involved in its achievement, since the user, the provider, and the financer of health care have different health, economic, and political interests. Quantifying the value chain's economic impact on society is relevant for its economic evaluation, reducing uncertainty and optimizing the design of public policies. There are theoretical and methodological weaknesses in the methods for estimating indirect costs of the value chain, including market imperfections and the postulates of economic theory.

The chapter designs the value chain for cervical cancer and the calculation of its costs, which is specified by highlighting the activities that contribute value to the disease's treatments and the activities considered to be supportive for the beneficiary of the treatments, that is, the patient.

Chapter 4, "Cytologic Monitoring, Management of Cervical Cancer, and Control of Human Papillomavirus" by Zakariyya Muhammad Bello discusses the role of cytologic monitoring, the management of cervical cancer, and the control of human papillomavirus (HPV) infections. Cervical cancer is the second most common cause of cancer-related death among women. It is caused by HPV, a double-stranded virus that leads to cellular alterations in the cervical squamocolumnar junction. Most HPV infections are cleared by the host immune system, while very few cases progress to invasive carcinoma due to persistent infection and other contributory risk factors. Several screening techniques have been devised over the years to detect HPV at an early stage, the most common being the Pap smear test, which can detect benign cellular changes and squamous intraepithelial neoplasias. Other important techniques involve visual inspection with acetic acid (VIA), colposcopy, and HPV DNA testing. In addition, recent advances have led to the development of new techniques such as biosensor and bioreceptor technology, and loop-mediated isothermal amplification (LAMP). Several methods have been in place to prevent the increased incidence of cervical cancer. Among these are prophylactic HPV vaccines, which elicit a humoral immune response against about 15 HPV genotypes. These vaccines do not cure established cancer, however. Several trials are underway to develop a therapeutic vaccine that will be effective in curing cervical cancer.

Michael Friedrich
Department of Obstetrics and Gynecology,
Helios Hospital,
Krefeld, Germany

Chapter 1

Molecular and Cell Biology of Cervical Cancer

Natalia Garcia-Becerra, Carlos A. Garcia-Becerra, Leonardo Fernandez-Avila, Jose Roberto Cruz-Lozano, Veronica Soltero-Molinar, Isabel Arias-Gallardo, Sofia Briseida Leyva-Delgado, Angel E. Chávez-Torres, Dalia I. Murillo-Geraldo and Jesús E. Juarez-Garcia

Abstract

The molecular and cell biology of cervical cancer will be covered in detail in this chapter, particularly emphasizing the disease's etiology, brief epidemiology, risk factors, cervical cancer hallmarks, and the main signaling pathways involved. The chapter will go in-depth about the characteristics of cancer, such as changes in cell cycle regulation, apoptosis, and cell differentiation, as well as the tumoral microenvironment. Signal pathways like the PI3K/AKT/mTOR pathway and the Wnt/beta-catenin pathway will be highlighted for their significance in the development of cervical cancer. The chapter will thoroughly explain the molecular and cell biology underlying this terrible illness.

Keywords: cervical cancer, molecular biology, cancer biology, cancer cells, tumor niche, tumor microenvironment, cancer signaling, hpv, cancer hallmarks

1. Introduction

Cervical cancer (CC) is a cellular alteration that originates in the cervix due to the persistent infection of oncogenic genotypes of the human papillomavirus (HPV) and initially manifests itself through precancerous lesions of slow and progressive evolution [1].

CC progression takes around 20 years to generate an invasive carcinoma; it begins with the precancerous lesions called cervical intraepithelial neoplasias (CIN) [2]. It is estimated that around 30% of women with advanced CIN premalignant lesions who do not receive treatment can progress to CC [3].

CC is recognized as a significant health burden in low- and middle-income countries, where it is ranked as the fourth most common type of female cancer [4, 5] and the second leading cause of cancer death in women worldwide [6]. In 2020, there were an estimated 604,000 new cases of cervical cancer and 324,000 deaths worldwide, with almost 90% of these cases occurring in low- and middle-income countries [6]. CC prevention is derived from vaccination schemes against HPV, the use of condoms, and timely detection of precancerous lesions through cervical cytology and HPV detection tests [7].

In October 2019, the World Health Organization (WHO) reported that 124 countries already had a timely and free vaccination program for 10-year-old girls. However, this is still insufficient to significantly reduce CC cases, given that the distribution of vaccines barely covers 30% of the world population, and screening schemes are not usually applied in all health sectors in low- and medium-income countries [8]. Because of this situation, in 2020, the WHO committee supported the Global Strategy towards the Elimination of Cervical Cancer, and it marked a significant milestone as it became the first-ever elimination strategy for a cancer in the history of the WHO.

The strategy sets forth three specific global targets aimed at preventing and treating CC; by 2030, 90% of girls should receive complete HPV vaccination before reaching 15 years of age; screening using a high-performance test should be conducted on 70% of women by age 35 and again by age 45; and 90% of identified CC patients should receive the suitable treatment [9]. These targets serve as measurable indicators to gauge progress in preventing and managing cervical cancer globally.

Known risk factors for developing CC are HPV, low socioeconomic status, smoking, young age at first intercourse, unprotected sexual intercourse, polygamy, long-term use of hormonal contraceptives, and multiple births [7, 10–13]. However, it has been shown that the most critical risk factor for CC development is persistent infection by high-risk HPV genotypes, which is essential for cell transformation and can be detected in 99.7% of CC cases [14, 15].

HPVs belong to the *Papillomaviridae* family, which are small, non-enveloped, double-stranded DNA viruses of about 50–60 nm diameter [16]. HPVs possess tropism for mucosal and cutaneous keratinocytes, and according to Papillomavirus Episteme, there are over two hundred genotypes that can be subclassified according to their oncogenic potential as high-risk and low-risk.

Low-risk HPVs, such as genotypes 6, 11, 42, 43, and 44, are classified as such because they commonly cause only benign epithelial lesions, such as warts and papillomas. On the other hand, high-risk genotypes, including 16, 18, 31, 33, 34, 39, 45, 52, 53, 58, 68, and 70, are strongly linked to the development of CC [17, 18]. Genotypes 16 and 18 are considered of the most significant clinical relevance due to their association with approximately 70% of the CC cases worldwide, in addition to their great oncogenic potential [19, 20].

The oncogenic nature of high-risk HPV is attributed to the activity of E6 and E7 oncoproteins, which are the only ones that remain active even when the transformation process of cervical cells has already begun [21]. Continuous expression of the E6 and E7 oncoproteins is essential to initiate and sustain the transformation of infected cells since they activate immunological and carcinogenic pathways to favor tumorigenesis and modulate local immunity [22, 23].

2. Oncogenes, tumor suppressor-genes, and mutations

Cancer develops due to a series of events at the molecular level triggered by genetic and epigenetic changes, which in turn modify the normal cellular biological behavior [24–26]. The molecular events are associated with the altered function of specific genes classified as proto-oncogenes and tumor suppressor genes (TSG); these maintain a balance among the normal cell life cycle, growth, and proliferation with programmed cell death (apoptosis) [26].

The transition from proto-oncogenes (genes with normal biological functions in cell homeostasis) to oncogenes (mutated proto-oncogenes with a gain in their normal biological function) is considered one of the first molecular events that trigger subsequent carcinogenesis [24, 25]. Changes in function from proto-oncogenes to oncogenes allow the appearance of key signs of cancer in a cell population, such as loss of apoptosis, uncontrolled cell multiplication, angiogenesis, and metastasis to distant organs [26].

Another fundamental molecular transformation for carcinogenesis is the loss of function of TSG, which is the primary antagonistic mechanism of carcinogenesis by maintaining cell homeostasis, promoting the repair of cell damage, and inducing apoptosis when this repair fails to occur [24, 26]; it has been hypothesized that the loss of function of both alleles of these genes is necessary to cause a phenotypic change; this is known as Knudson's phenomenon or the "two-hit theory" [27].

2.1 Cervical cancer and tumor suppressor genes

A sequence of steps in carcinogenesis onset related to high-risk HPV has been hypothesized in CC, presumably beginning with the decrease in the activity of tumor suppressor genes [26].

HPV infects the basal cells of the cervical epithelium, using the normal cycle of epithelial cells, which replicate in the basal region (where the virus replicates minimally), migrate to the apical region, and specialize (where viral replication increases) [28–30]. The process of carcinogenesis secondary to infection entails a process of several decades of persistent or repetitive infection, in which, also accidentally, the viral genome integrates into the host genome [26, 28, 30, 31], which is not part of the normal life cycle of the virus [30].

Upon integration into the genome, various molecular processes take place. These processes have two outcomes: Firstly, they interfere with the *E2* gene from inhibiting the *E6* and *E7* viral oncogenes [32, 33], and secondly, they contribute to an increase in genomic instability of neighboring sections of the host DNA. This instability is caused by mechanisms such as insertion into fragile regions, rearrangement or duplication of contiguous genes, and the specific way viral genes are inserted [30, 31, 34]. Regarding TSG, E6 induces ubiquitin-mediated degradation of p53 protein, so its protective action against genetic damage is inhibited [22, 28]; E7 interacts with the LXCXE motif segment of the amino-terminal end of the Rb family of proteins (Rb, p110, p130, and p107 mainly), suppressing them and allowing the unopposed expression of E2F transcription factor, progressing from G1 to S phase in the cell cycle (**Figure 1**) [22, 28].

2.2 Proto-oncogenes and oncogenes

Once genomic instability and cell immortalization are established by mechanisms that will be described further, it is considered that oncogenesis continues with the transition from proto-oncogenes to oncogenes. One of the main pathways described in more than 90% of cells with CC is mediated by PI3K/Akt [35], which promotes mechanisms of cellular proliferation; the activation of this pathway has been described secondary to the suppression of the PTEN gene [35] or to the overexpression of PI3KCA [25].

Other important oncogenes related to the proliferation of CC are the *c-myc* transcription factor, the *ERB2* tyrosine kinase receptor, and the "*HaRAS*" oncogene [35].

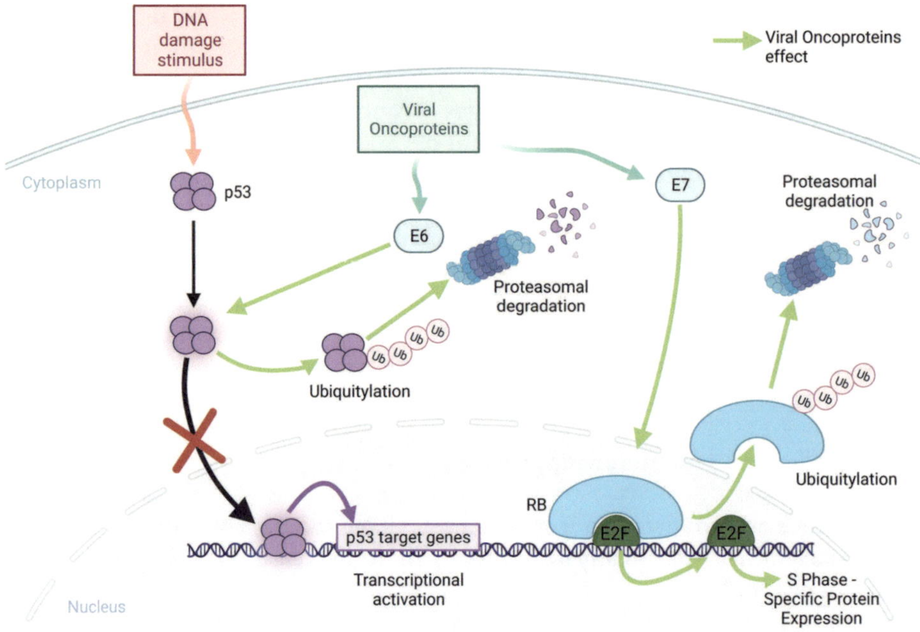

Figure 1.
Schematic representation of the main action of E6 and E7 viral oncoproteins on tumor suppressor genes. E6 blocking the function of the tp53 protein and inducing its degradation. E7 blocking the function of the RB protein and inducing its degradation.

3. Cell survival and immortality in cervical cancer

In CC, cancer cells survive by avoiding apoptosis and acquiring the capacity to replicate indefinitely. These characteristics and other hallmarks of cancer allow its uncontrolled proliferation and the formation of tumor masses in the cervix [36]. *Apoptosis* is a crucial physiological mechanism that limits the expansion of the cell population, to maintain tissue homeostasis by eliminating aged cells or cells that have outlived their useful life and allowing cell renewal or by eliminating potentially malignant cells that are experiencing irreparable damage caused by internal or external factors [37].

It is thus a well-recognized fact that resistance to apoptosis is a hallmark of cancer in general, a requirement for the persistence of transformed cells that, through various strategies, manage to evade it [36].

Nevertheless, what allows CC cells to overcome apoptosis? Aforesaid, HPV infection is a necessary and predisposing factor for developing and progressing CC. Interestingly, HPV E6 and E7 oncoproteins have been shown to enable cancer cells to escape apoptosis by disrupting or modifying pathways that precipitate this mechanism and that are finely regulated by pro- and anti-apoptotic proteins [38]. The ubiquitin-mediated degradation of p53 by E6 oncoprotein prevents cell cycle arrest and, ultimately, the apoptotic machinery, mediated in part by transcriptional activation of BAX and PUMA [39]. Given this fact, it is worth mentioning that the presence of E6 leads to a significant increase in the activity of the *survivin* promoter, a protein that prevents apoptosis. *Survivin* expression is negatively regulated by p53, and since E6 negatively regulates p53, it is likely that it also influences the regulation of *survivin* transcription. This suggests that the *survivin* gene is relevant to the anti-apoptotic function of E6. In addition, E6 can also bind directly to BAK protein, causing its degradation, thus blocking the intrinsic or mitochondrial pathway of apoptosis. The binding capacity of E6 to this protein is similar in HPVs considered high or low risk, suggesting that the inactivation of BAK is essential for the virus replication cycle [40]. E6 also prevents an extrinsic receptor-mediated response to apoptosis. *In vitro* studies have shown that E6 protein protects cells from TNF-mediated death through a p53-independent mechanism. It has been observed that E6 binds to a specific part of the TNF-R1 receptor, preventing apoptotic signal transduction [41]. Likewise, it has been pointed out that E6 can bind to the DED domains of the adaptor protein FADD and pro-caspase 8, critical elements of the extrinsic pathway, stimulating their degradation [42]. These findings show that E6 promotes survival by exerting multiple effects that inhibit apoptosis.

Regarding E7 oncoprotein, its role in cell cycle has been previously described; however, concerning apoptosis, it plays a dual role; it can induce or inhibit this process depending on its interaction with different proteins and mechanisms and significantly depending on the HPV present [43].

Moreover, considering that the E5 oncoprotein does not usually receive much attention due to its elimination at later stages of infection, it is essential to mention that its presence in early stages is crucial for survival and propagation of the virus in the cervical epithelium [44]. It modulates the epidermal growth factor signaling pathway, which induces the degradation of BAX, which is essential for triggering the intrinsic apoptosis pathway [45]. A relationship has also been found between its presence and the downregulation of death receptors such as CD95 in cervical tumors leading to impaired apoptosis [46].

Given that CC cells have effectively evaded the apoptosis mechanism, it is essential to mention that this enables them to achieve immortality, that is, an unlimited replication potential, thus contributing to the development and progression of cancer. Usually, as cells replicate, the ends of the chromosomes that protect the DNA during cell division, called telomeres, shorten with each successive cycle. This is part of cellular aging. However, in cancer cells, it is necessary to prevent the telomeres from shortening so the tumor can continue growing [47].

Telomerase is an enzyme responsible for telomere replication and is overexpressed in cancer cells but inactive in healthy cells [48]. In this regard, it has already been reported that HPV E6 and E7 persistently drive the expression of a catalytic unit in telomerase called hTERT, which gives these cells unlimited replicative capacity [49]. This is possible because E6 and E7 activate the hTERT promoter with the help of proteins such as c-myc and Sp1 that act as positive regulators and NFX1. NFX1 normally represses hTERT expression but is degraded by E6/E6AP, which activates the hTERT promoter [50].

4. Main signaling pathways (JAK/STAT, Ras/MEK/Erk, PI3K/Akt/mTOR, WNT/b-catenin)

Giving continuity to the critical regulation of external and internal factors on cell function, space is given to understand the signaling that makes this possible at the molecular level. Below are four signaling pathways relevant to the development of CC since their inappropriate regulation allows the cell to experience anabolic, proliferative, growth-promoting, and cell-survival effects.

4.1 Janus Kinase/Signal Transducer and Transcription Activator (JAK/STAT) signaling pathway

The Janus Kinase/Signal Transducer and Transcription Activator (JAK/STAT) signaling pathway is characterized by its physiological contribution to cell proliferation, differentiation, and death by causing a final gene transcription reaction in the cell nucleus. Its dysfunction can cause alterations in immune regulation and tumor processes [51].

The sequence of events begins with the interaction of cytokines and growth factors with their respective receptors, types I and II, on the cell membrane. The intracellular portion of the receptor interacts with the inactive JAK [52], which undergoes dimerization and oligomerization [53]. In both cases, a conformational change is induced in the cytoplasmic domain [52]. The described effect is the juxtaposition of JAKs for their phosphorylation and transphosphorylation by other JAKs or other families of tyrosine kinases.

Activation of JAKs phosphorylates the cytoplasmic domain, creating a binding site for other signaling molecules such as STAT proteins [51]. Cytoplasmic STAT binds to phosphorylated receptors, thus becoming substrates to be phosphorylated by JAKs. After phosphorylation, STATs form homodimers or heterodimers capable of translocating to the nucleus and activating gene transcription [23, 51]. Regulators of this pathway have been identified as suppressor signaling cytokines (SOCS), activated protein inhibitors of STAT (PIAS), and protein tyrosine phosphatases (PTP) [54].

4.2 Mitogen-activated protein kinase (MAPK) signaling pathway

Similarly, the dysfunction and incorrect regulation of the mitogen-activated protein kinase (MAPK) signaling cascade has been linked to carcinogenic events since it is also involved in cell proliferation, survival, differentiation, and migration [55, 56]. This cascade begins with stimuli, including growth factors, tumor-promoting substances, and differentiation factors. There is a stimulation of Ras-GDP to convert to Ras-GTP, resulting in its activation resulting in its activation and subsequent Raf phosphorylation. In turn, Raf is responsible for the phosphorylation of MEK1. MEK1 phosphorylates ERK, an extracellular receptor kinase responsible for regulating cytosolic proteins, transcription factors, and metastasis [55, 56].

4.3 PI3K/AKT/mTOR signaling cascade

The PI3K/AKT/mTOR signaling cascade also affects energy metabolism. The negative effects related to CC lie in the contribution to the creation and proliferation of malignant cell phenotypes [55, 56]. The cascade begins with a lipid kinase, PI3K, activated by the effect of extracellular stimuli recognized by receptors associated with G proteins (GPCRs) or receptor tyrosine kinases (RTKs), also using Ras-GTPases [55, 56]. The stimuli in question are given by growth factors or cytokines, which cause receptor dimerization and transphosphorylation. Once the receptor is phosphorylated, it is ready to bind to and activate proteins, in this case, PI3K. Activated PI3K produces PIP3, from PIP2, and PI(3,4)P2. PIP3, in turn, attracts the AKT molecule to the cell membrane, which is then phosphorylated and activated by PDK1 and mTORC2 [57]. AKT is responsible for activating mTORC1, the molecule responsible for the anabolic effects in the cell. This signaling cascade is important in regulating cell functions such as cell growth, motility, survival, metabolism, and angiogenesis [55, 56]. Dysfunction of this cascade, particularly its overactivation, is implicated in carcinogenesis.

4.4 WNT/beta-catenin signaling pathway

Lastly, the fourth relevant signaling pathway in the pathogenesis of CC is Wnt/beta-catenin, also called canonical. Wnt is proteins incorporated into exosomes for transport and have target-specific genes that can be transcribed through beta-catenin stabilization [58]. Beta-catenin in its inactive state is bound to the so-called destruction complex consisting of Axin, CKI, GSK3, APC, Dvl (or Dsh), and Beta-TrCP (**Figure 2**), which regulates it by degradation [59]. Beta-catenin phosphorylation serves as a stimulus for beta-TrCP to ubiquitinate it, resulting in its proteasomal. The effects of beta-catenin can be evidenced only by avoiding its degradation when its levels in the cytosol are high.

The beginning of the cascade occurs when Wnt activates its receptor complex formed by the Frizzled receptor and co-receptor LRP5/6; this induces the phosphorylation of LRP6 by CK1 and GSK3, allowing the translocation of the destruction complex from the cytosol to the membrane [58]. This process activates the Dvl (Dsh) component, which in its active state induces the sequestration or degradation of Axin in such a way that it inhibits the destruction complex by stabilizing cytosolic beta-catenin [59]. Wnt has target genes within the DNA in the nucleus and requires a molecule called TCF for its transcription. In the inactive Wnt state, TCF in the nucleus is inhibited by Groucho, preventing it from binding to DNA and starting gene transcription [60, 61]. In its active state, Wnt triggers the steps mentioned above, culminating in the increase in intracellular beta-catenin. As beta-catenin accumulates

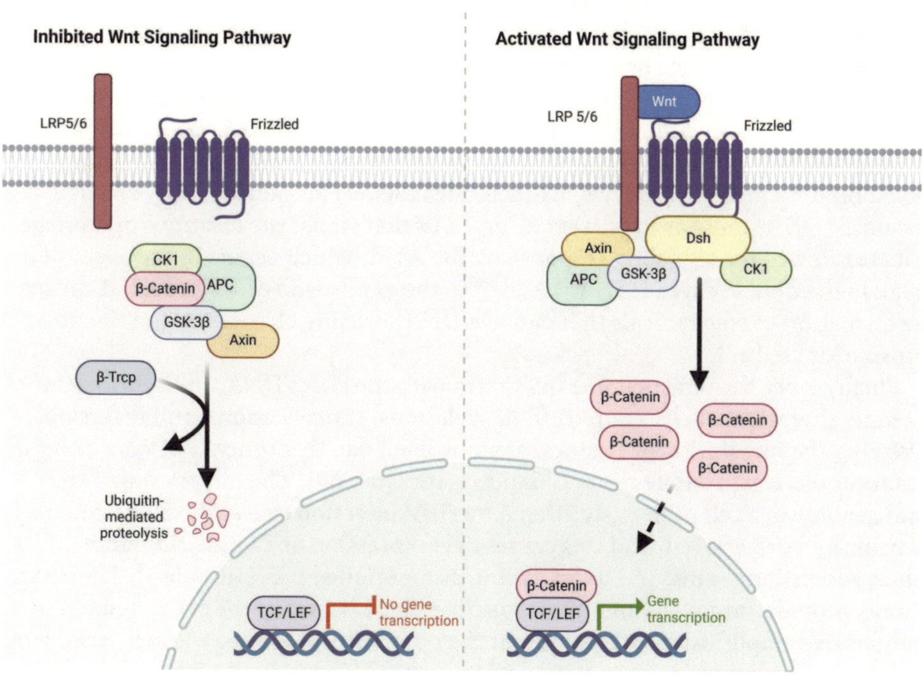

Figure 2.
Schematic representation of the molecular components taking part in the Wnt/beta-catenin pathway.

in the cytosol, it enters the nucleus, removes Groucho from its inhibitory position, and binds to TCF [60, 61]. This accumulation leads to the transcription of Wnt target genes. The effects of Wnt/beta-catenin signaling in CC promote epithelial-mesenchymal transition, migration, growth, and cell proliferation [62].

The beginning of the cascade occurs when Wnt activates its receptor complex formed by the Frizzled receptor and co-receptor LRP5/6; this induces the phosphorylation of LRP6 by CK1 and GSK3, allowing the translocation of the destruction complex from the cytosol to the membrane [58]. This process activates the Dvl (Dsh) component, which in its active state induces the sequestration or degradation of Axin in such a way that it inhibits the destruction complex by stabilizing cytosolic beta-catenin [59]. Wnt has target genes within the DNA in the nucleus and requires a molecule called TCF for its transcription. In the inactive Wnt state, TCF in the nucleus is inhibited by Groucho, preventing it from binding to DNA and starting gene transcription [60, 61]. In its active state, Wnt triggers the steps mentioned above, culminating in the increase in intracellular beta-catenin. As beta-catenin accumulates in the cytosol, it enters the nucleus, removes Groucho from its inhibitory position, and binds to TCF [60, 61].

This accumulation leads to the transcription of Wnt target genes. The effects of Wnt/beta-catenin signaling in CC promote epithelial-mesenchymal transition, migration, growth, and cell proliferation [62].

5. Cell cycle alterations and genomic instability

Viral infections are related to about 9.9% of cancers worldwide as they contribute to the oncogenesis of host cells [63]. The transformative process of the HPV-infected cell could be classified as a multifactorial process in its virulence mechanisms, which ensure the survival and proliferation of the virus at the expense of the integrity of the human genome, implying a loss of genomic stability through a mutation or an oncogenic exposure, thus being the center point of cancer [36].

The intrinsic HPV proteins that are especially important in the transformative process of the cell are initially the E1 and E2 proteins and the E6 and E7 [64]. The process begins with the integration of the viral genome through the E1 helicase and the E2 binding protein; likewise, E1 facilitates the recruitment of DNA damage response (DDR) mechanisms, a set of proteins that signal the locations of damage to its repair and the signaling response by the ATM, which occurs in the event of a break in the double chain [65, 66]. Added to the expression of E1 and E2, it causes the formation of free radicals that damage DNA, causing changes in guanine to tyrosine kinase [67].

Finally, once the viral genome integrates with the host's DNA, the hybrid gene presents alterations such as duplications, deletions, translocations, and inversions. Likewise, the integration of the viral genome itself can theoretically act as a *de novo* mutation and can promote recombination errors [64, 68]. The integration of the viral genome in a cell previously altered by HPV infection causes the E2 protein to be truncated or removed, and this causes overexpression of E6 and, therefore, of its genes, which derives into p53 degradation, as mentioned previously [64]. The E6 and E7 oncoproteins target p53 and Rb, respectively, predisposing the cell to remain in the proliferative amplification stage without the possibility of exiting the cell cycle, which leads to the accumulation of mutations. However, E7 individually can transform a cell into a cancer cell [69].

Ubiquitin-mediated degradation of p53 by E6 promotes genomic instability and the subsequent birth of cancer [64], since the absence of p53 activity allows the cell to proceed to the S phase of the cell cycle without having repaired the damaged areas of the DNA [21].

The progression from G1 to S without previous DNA revision and repair results in the accumulation of errors in the chromosomes [64]. E7 is the primary mediator for DDR activation, which is localized to the junction foci of the viral genome with the host genome. It is theorized that this DDR hijacking prevents the repair of further DNA damage [70]. In response to DDR, targeted transduction of the viral genome mediated by homologous recombination reduces the capacity to repair DNA double-strand breaks by 50% [71].

Other pro-carcinogenic activities of the E6 and E7 oncoproteins are the association with centrosome amplification and shortening, increasing cell cycle defects [71, 72]. This process drives the proliferation of infected cells from infected keratinocytes [22, 73]. The effect of E6 and E7 on telomeres causes lengthening and sometimes shortening capable of driving arrangements such as bridging in anaphase and "breakage-fusion-bridge" cycles or replication indefinitely [64, 74]; in CC, 64% of the cases show a high expression of alteration in telomeres [64, 75].

6. Metabolic switch

The "metabolic switch" or deregulation of cellular metabolism is considered one of the hallmarks of cancer and refers to the metabolic mutation that tumor cells present with an affinity for "aerobic" glycolysis to obtain energy and favor the synthesis of macromolecules for the cellular replacement [76–78], which will be explained in detail later.

Under normal conditions, healthy body cells in the presence of oxygen obtain energy through aerobic metabolism, that is, the citric acid cycle or Krebs cycle, where carbohydrates, amino acids, and lipids are metabolized [77]. Due to the oxidations in this cycle, three molecules of nicotinamide adenine dinucleotide (NAD) and one of flavin adenine dinucleotide (FAD) are produced (generating 2.5 ATP each NADH and 1.5 ATP each FADH) [77]. Those molecules (NADH and FADH) subsequently enter the respiratory chain and oxidative phosphorylation, resulting in a total of up to 36 ATP molecules through these aerobic routes [77].

Additionally, there is glycolysis, a metabolic pathway that occurs in normal cells without oxygen, where glucose is catabolized, obtaining 2 ATP molecules and two pyruvate molecules for each glucose molecule [79]. Both routes end with the same goal: to satisfy the energy needs of the tissues.

Most malignant cells alter these metabolic pathways to obtain energy (**Figure 3**), presenting greater glucose uptake compared to normal cells and metabolizing it through glycolysis, most of which is converted into lactate even in the presence of a high oxygen level. This metabolic deregulation is known as the Warburg Effect, where Otto Warburg postulated that malignant cells obtained their energy from "aerobic" glycolysis [76]. This restructuring favors and fosters an environment suitable for the use of cancer cells [76, 78]. Although glycolysis is less efficient to produce enough ATP molecules, cancer cells alter metabolic pathways using glycolysis as the main pathway and oxidative phosphorylation to a lesser extent, resulting in a fast production of ATP to meet the exuberant energy demands of cancer cells during their proliferation [80].

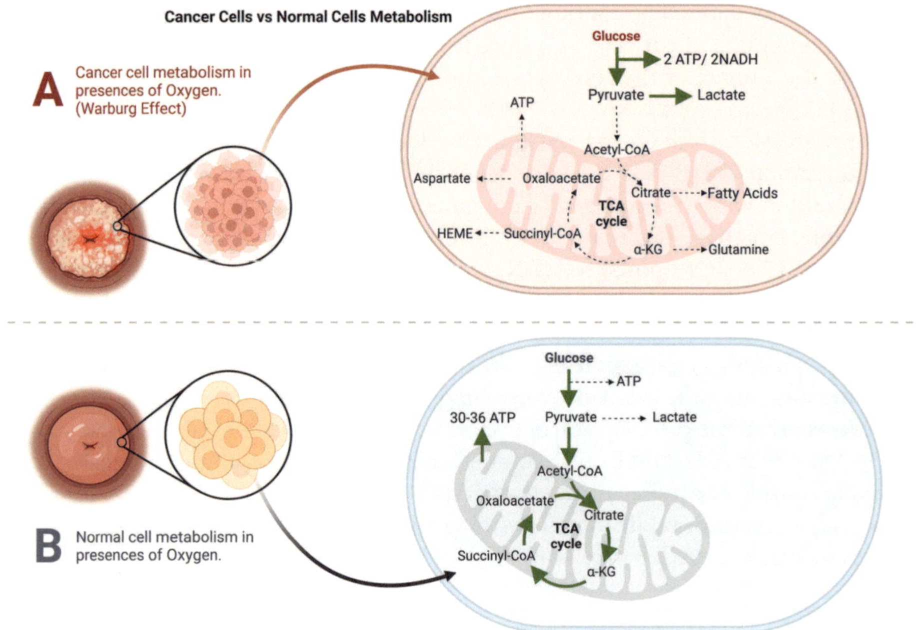

Figure 3.
Comparison of cancer cell metabolism vs. normal cell metabolism, both in the presence of oxygen.

In glycolysis, there is a leak of substrates useful for other metabolic routes with intermediate products that will serve for the subsequent synthesis of proteins, nucleic acids, and lipids that are fundamental for the development and division of malignant cells [81, 82]. In turn, this dysregulation prompts cellular adaptation to metabolic stress and protects cancer cells from reactive oxygen species (ROS)-related damage [82].

The specific role of HPV occurs in the microenvironment after the infection by this virus helps to evade the immune response and promote local immunosuppression [80]; in addition, it contributes to the restructuring of the metabolism of infected cells in the immune microenvironment. There is evidence of metabolism changes related to glutamine, taurine, and lysine in positive cases of HPV, which are related to the interaction of this pathogen and normal cellular metabolism [83]. Also, E6 and E7 may favor the Warburg effect by contributing to chemoresistance [29, 84].

When lactate accumulates in abnormal cells, the acid environment facilitates the deregulation of normal metabolism and signaling pathways of immune cells such as dendritic cells, macrophages, and T lymphocytes, producing the immune response. While all these changes are favorable to continue viral propagation and the persistence of the malignant cellular process, T lymphocytes are forced to change by such a high lactate environment, decreasing their functionality [80].

7. Cervical cancer and immune system

CC has two essential elements for its establishment and progression: the parenchyma, comprised of cancer cells, and the stroma, which includes connective tissue, blood vessels, extracellular matrix (ECM), nutrients, and the immune system [77]. These elements contribute through three situations: immune escaping, angiogenesis activation, and tumor progression (proliferation, invasion, and metastasis) [85].

The tumor microenvironment (TME) is defined as a complex ecosystem surrounding a tumor inside the body; the TME is in a constant battle between a tumor suppression response and a tumor-promoting response [86].

Cancer cells represent the core of the TME, and they are responsible for manipulating the cell and non-cell components through signaling mechanisms to take advantage of the non-tumoral cells to promote carcinogenesis and metastasis [87].

Intercellular communication is generated by the synthesis of cytokines, chemokines, growth factors, and inflammatory mediators, among others, but novel mechanisms recently reported include cell-free DNA, exosomes, circulating tumor cells, and apoptotic bodies [88–91].

Near the tumoral cell core, cancer-associated fibroblasts (CAFs) are located; these populations play a crucial role in carcinogenesis as they promote the proliferation, migration, and survival of cancer cells [91]; however, it is essential to acknowledge that as a heterogeneous cell population, some are related to antitumoral activities. In the tumoral niche, some CAFs promote the recruitment of immunosuppressive cells through the synthesis of ECM proteins [92], and others promote angiogenesis by producing fibroblast growth factor 2 (FGF2) and vascular endothelial growth factor A (VEGFA); they also offer nutrients to tumoral cells such as ketone and cytokines necessary for mitochondrial biogenesis and autophagy [93].

Among the non-malignant cells located at TME are the tumor-infiltrating lymphocytes (TILs), which comprise one of the primary mediators of the dynamic yet ambiguous immune response. This group comprises T cell subsets such as CD4+, CD8+, regulatory T cells (Tregs), and Natural Killer (NK) cells [94]. Even though most of these cell populations are specialized in antitumoral functions, the overall action is insufficient to eradicate the tumor effectively due to the low levels of antitumoral cells, and the TME promotes an immuno-suppressor stimulus that induces a senescent state among those cells. In CC, the presence of cytotoxic CD8+ T cells activated by tumoral antigens is recognized as an excellent prognostic marker due to their killing activities and suppression of angiogenesis through IL-2 and IFN-γ secretion. On the other hand, CD4+ T cells coordinate an ambiguous immune response; Th1 cells synthesize potent modulators of cell-mediated immune responses [95]. However, recent studies have demonstrated that CIN or CC patients had a lower proportion of Th1 subtype and a higher proportion of Th2, Th17, and Treg cells when compared against healthy controls, and this imbalance aggravates along with the progression of the disease [96].

Finally, it is essential to mention the role of macrophages since they represent one of the significant components of tumor infiltrates and are responsible for producing high amounts of inflammatory molecules, IL-1β, IL-6, IL-23, and TNF-α, ROS, hypoxia-induced factor (HIF), necessary for inflammatory processes [97]. At the TME, macrophages are identified as Tumor-Associated Macrophages (TAMs) and are often associated with tumor progression and worsening of CC patients. TAMs can polarize into two phenotypes, M1 macrophages that release inflammatory factors, promote immune responses, and inhibit the CC occurrence [98], and the M2 phenotype, which is correlated with poor prognosis, chemoresistance, and diminished patient survival [99].

The growing evidence demonstrates the relevance of the TME in CC progression since the interaction between tumoral cells and their surroundings promotes their proliferation, resistance to apoptosis, chemoresistance, aggressiveness, and immune evasion. Thus, TME is crucial in determining CC patients' therapeutic response and clinical outlook.

8. Angiogenesis

Angiogenesis is the formation of new blood vessels as an essential mechanism for the growth, survival, and spread of solid tumors [100]. This process not only occurs in neoplasias but also is involved in the growth of the endometrium and fetal development, among other processes [101, 102].

For the formation of new vessels, in tumor development, there is an imbalance between stimulating and inhibitory factors, where there is an increase in angiogenic factors such as vascular endothelial growth factor (VEGF), fibroblast growth factor (FGF), platelet-derived growth factor (PDGF), and angiopoietins (Ang), which are produced by the same tumor cells, macrophages, and lymphocytes that may be attached to the tumor [103, 104]. In addition, a decrease in antiangiogenic agents such as Thrombospodin-1 (TSP-1) is detected, allowing the transition from an avascular phase to a vascular phase, also called "angiogenic switch" [105–107].

This imbalance begins in the tumor cells, where there are areas with little irrigation and, therefore, low oxygenation; this tumoral tissue starts producing HIF1, which is a regulator of the recruitment of endothelial progenitor cells (EPC), pericyte progenitor cells (PPC), and monocytes, and thus carries out vascular restructuring; it also increases VEGF activity [108–110].

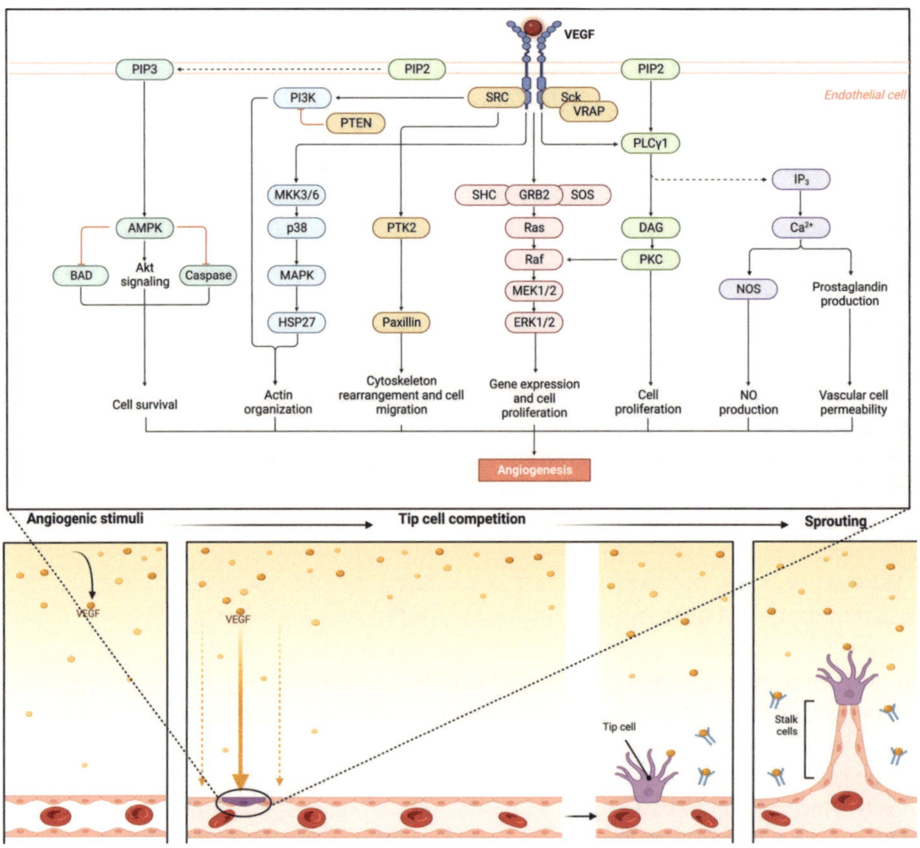

Figure 4.
Schematic representation of the intracellular response to VEGF stimulation, in tumor angiogenesis.

VEGF, the major angiogenic factor, consists of a family of proteins, VEGF-A, VEGF-B, VEGF-C, VEGF-D, VEGF-E, and the placental growth factor. These proteins interact with three tyrosine kinase receptors, with VEGFR1 and VEGFR2, to trigger the signaling cascade promoting migration, proliferation, and survival of endothelial cells, also increasing the permeability of existing blood vessels, and this allows the leakage of multiple plasma proteins and the formation of new vessels (**Figure 4**). VEGF also inhibits apoptosis of newly formed blood vessels [111, 112].

FGF-1 and FGF-2 are also important angiogenic factors; FGF-2 increases the expression of other angiogenic agents, such as VEGF, and regulates the balance of Ang, leading to a predominance of Ang-2 [113–115]. On the other hand, Ang-2 is secreted by endothelial cells at sites of active vascular remodeling and engages in tumor initiation. Multiple studies indicate that the imbalance of Ang-2 and Ang-1 is associated with vascular instability, a key point in the initiation of angiogenesis in tumors [115, 116].

In recent years, efforts have been made to inhibit the signaling cascade in CC as a possible therapeutic target. There are several drugs in use, such as bevacizumab, which is a drug that inhibits the formation of new vessels by neutralizing VEGF activity, among others. However, these drugs must be in conjunction with chemotherapy or radiation therapy [117–120].

9. Epithelial-mesenchymal transition & metastasis

As the fourth most common cancer among females worldwide, lymph node metastasis (LNM) is a key prognostic factor and a leading cause of death in patients with CC [121]. In metastasis, the ability to undergo reversible cellular and phenotypic changes is crucial for disseminating cancer cells to adapt to the changing microenvironments and stress during this pathological process. One main form of cellular plasticity is the epithelial-mesenchymal transition (EMT); in this process, epithelial cells lose tight cell-cell connections and polarity, which confers migratory and invasive properties (**Figure 5**); in its reverse process, mesenchymal-epithelial transition (MET) cells loose migratory freedom; they begin expressing junction complexes and adopt apicobasal polarity. This form of cellular plasticity may occur in physiological processes like human embryonic development (e.g., neural crest formation) and pathological conditions such as organ fibrosis, cancer progression, and metastasis [122, 123].

9.1 Metastasis cascade

Tumor cells that have undergone EMT exhibit stem-cell-like properties, including the ability to self-renew, tumor-initiation properties, and resistance to chemotherapy and radiotherapy, which explains why metastasis is the primary cause of death in cancer patients and why advances in tumor expression markers can help identify and prevent metastasis from happening [123, 124].

There are different markers to identify the state in which a tumor cell can be found; in the case of tumor cells in the epithelial state, researchers look out for the expression of E-cadherin, EpCAM, claudins, occludins, and cytokeratins; in the case of cells in the mesenchymal state, they can look for expression of vimentin (VIM), fibronectin, and α-SMA [125].

While EMT does not require changes in DNA sequence and can be reversible [124], the same cannot be said about other pathways; for example, due to high energy demand

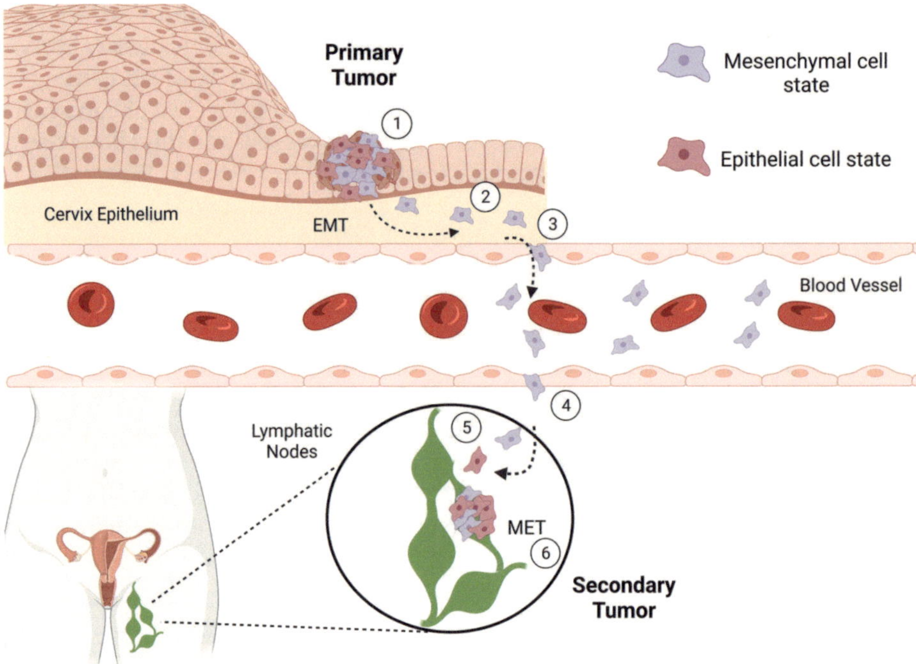

Figure 5.
Stepwise epithelial-mesenchymal transitions. 1. Tumor cells acquire the ability to dissociate themselves from the primary tumor mass through EMT; these epithelial cells lose their cell-cell junctions to become motile. 2. Now these cells can migrate and invade through the ECM. 3. Intravasation into blood vessels or lymphatic vessels occur; in this phase, tumor cells pass through the endothelial lamina and enter systemic circulation. 4. During extravasation, tumor cells extravasate through the capillary endothelium of distant organs into its parenchyma. 5. Tumor cells establish themselves and proliferate, forming micrometastases. 6. Colonization of distant organs and re-activation of epithelial properties occur at the secondary site via the MET where these cells become malignant secondary tumors; EMT facilitates cancer cells to invade, intravasate, and survive in circulation; cancer cells need to undergo MET to colonize efficiently at distant organs.

during EMT, several morphological and metabolic changes are made by 5’AMP-activated kinase (AMPK), which is a cellular energy homeostasis sensor that controls the balance between energy intake and demand; it modulates processes such as carbohydrate and lipid metabolism, biosynthesis, autophagy, and cell cycle.

Specifically, in the case of CC metastasis, a study by Konieczny et al. demonstrated that AMPK expression is related to malignant behavior in CC cells [126]. Another example is the case of protein tyrosine phosphatase receptor type M (PTPRM); Liu et al. demonstrated that PTPRM was upregulated in CC with LNM; as a result, it promoted tumor cell proliferation, migration, and lymphangiogenesis (a critical early metastasis event important in LNM and a prognosis factor in patients with cervical cancer), as well as EMT *via* the activation of Src-AKT signaling pathway and induced lymphangiogenesis in a VEGF-C-dependent manner [121]. Research on the EMT and MET has also uncovered numerous novel signaling pathways, including TGF-β, Wnt, Notch, Hedgehog, and PI3K pathways, that facilitate EMT in tumor cells [121].

10. Conclusion

In the previous chapter, the currently known mechanisms that promote CC oncogenesis were explained. It is essential to emphasize the evident relationship between infection by high-risk HPV serotypes and the development of CC. There are well-defined molecular mechanisms by years of research since the relationship was discovered by Zur Hausen et al. regarding CC and HPV. Although there are still other mechanisms pending elucidation, what is clear is that the more its etiopathogenesis and the complexity of its molecular mechanics are known, the more are the possibilities of developing effective treatments.

Appendices and nomenclature

ADC	adenocarcinoma
ADSC	adenosquamous carcinoma
AMPK	5'AMP-activated kinase
Ang	angiopoietins
CC	cervical cancer
CIN	cervical intraepithelial neoplasia
DDR	DNA damage response
EMC	extracellular matrix
EMT	epithelial-mesenchymal transition
EPC	endothelial progenitor cells
FAD	flavin adenine dinucleotide
GFGF	fibroblast growth factor
GPCR	receptors associated with G protein.
HIF-1	hypoxia-induced factor-1
HPV	human papillomavirus
hTERT	human telomerase reverse transcriptase
JAK/STAT	janus kinase/ signal transducer and transcription activator
LMN	lymph node metastasis
MAPK	mitogen activated protein kinase
MET	mesenchymal-epithelial transition
NAD	nicotinamide adenine dinucleotide
PDGF	platelet-derived growth factor
PIAS	activated protein inhibitors of stat.
PPC	pericyte progenitor cells
PTP	protein tyrosine phosphatase
PTPRM	protein tyrosine phosphatase receptor type M
ROS	reactive oxygen species
RTKs	receptor tyrosine kinase
SCC	squamous cell carcinoma
SOCS	suppressor signaling cytokines.
TAM	tumor-associated macrophages
TILs	tumor-infiltrating lymphocytes
TME	tumor microenvironment
Tregs	regulatory T cells
TSG	tumor suppressor genes
TSP-1	Thrombospondin-1
VEGF	vascular endothelial growth factor
VIM	vimentin
WHO	World Health Organization

Author details

Natalia Garcia-Becerra[1*], Carlos A. Garcia-Becerra[2], Leonardo Fernandez-Avila[1], Jose Roberto Cruz-Lozano[1], Veronica Soltero-Molinar[2], Isabel Arias-Gallardo[1], Sofia Briseida Leyva-Delgado[3], Angel E. Chávez-Torres[1], Dalia I. Murillo-Geraldo[2] and Jesús E. Juarez-Garcia[2]

1 UdeG, Guadalajara, Mexico

2 UAG, Guadalajara, Mexico

3 UMSNH, Morelia, Mexico

*Address all correspondence to: nat.garciab96@gmail.com

References

[1] Sanchez Gaitan E. Tamizaje y tratamiento de las lesiones precancerosas para la prevención del cáncer cervicouterino. Revista Medica Sinergia. 2019;**4**:e300. DOI: 10.31434/rms.v4i11.300

[2] Prendiville W, Sankaranarayanan R. Colposcopy and Treatment of Cervical Precancer. Vol. 45. Lyon, France: World Health Organization; 2017. p. 178

[3] Eun T, Perkins J. Screening for cervical cancer. Medical Clinics of North America. 2020;**104**:15. DOI: 10.1016/j.mcna.2020.08.006

[4] Buskwofie A, David-West G, Clare CA. A review of cervical cancer: Incidence and disparities. Journal of the National Medical Association. 2020;**112**:229-232. DOI: 10.1016/j.jnma.2020.03.002

[5] Arbyn M, Weiderpass E, Bruni L, de Sanjosé S, Saraiya M, Ferlay J, et al. Estimates of incidence and mortality of cervical cancer in 2018: A worldwide analysis. The Lancet Global Health. 2020;**8**:e191-e203. DOI: 10.1016/s2214-109x(19)30482-6

[6] Sung H, Ferlay J, Siegel RL, Laversanne M, Soerjomataram I, Jemal A, et al. Global cancer statistics 2020: GLOBOCAN estimates of incidence and mortality worldwide for 36 cancers in 185 countries. CA: A Cancer Journal for Clinicians. 2021;**71**:209-249. DOI: 10.3322/caac.21660

[7] Zhang S, Huifang X, Zhang L, Qiao Y. Cervical cancer: Epidemiology, risk factors and screening. Chinese Journal of Cancer Research. 2020;**32**:8

[8] Organization, W.H. Major Milestone Reached as 100 Countries have Introduced HPV Vaccine into National Schedule. Available from: https://www.who.int/news/item/31-10-2019-major-milestone-reached-as-100-countries-have-introduced-hpv-vaccine-into-national-schedule

[9] Organization PAH. Pan American Health Organization. Plan of Action for Cervical Cancer Prevention and Control 2018-2030. Washington, D.C.: PAHO; 2018. pp. 1-44

[10] Kuhn L, Denny L, Pollack A, Lorincz A, Richart R, Wright T. Human papillomavirus DNA testing for cervical cancer screening in low-resource settings. Journal of the National Center Institute. 2000;**92**:7. DOI: 10.1093/jnci/92.10.818

[11] Hellberg D. Sex steroids and cervical cancer. Anticancer Research. 2012;**32**:9

[12] Fonseca-Moutinho J. Smoking and cervical cancer. ISRN Obstetrics and Gynecology. 2011;**2011**:1-6

[13] Jensen KE, Schmiedel S, Norrild B, Frederiksen K, Iftner T, Kjaer SK. Parity as a cofactor for high-grade cervical disease among women with persistent human papillomavirus infection: A 13-year follow-up. British Journal of Cancer. 2013;**108**:234-239. DOI: 10.1038/bjc.2012.513

[14] Kashyap N, Krishnan N, Kaur S, Ghai S. Risk factors of cervical cancer: A case-control study. Asia-Pacific Journal of Oncology Nursing. 2019;**6**:308-314. DOI: 10.4103/apjon.apjon_73_18

[15] Ngoma M, Autier P. Cancer prevention: Cervical cancer. Ecancermedicalscience. 2019;**13**:952. DOI: 10.3332/ecancer.2019.952

[16] Harden ME, Munger K. Human papillomavirus molecular biology.

Mutation Research, Reviews in Mutation Research. 2017;**772**:3-12. DOI: 10.1016/j.mrrev.2016.07.002

[17] Leite KRM, Pimenta R, Canavez J, Canavez F, de Souza FR, Vara L, et al. HPV genotype prevalence and success of vaccination to prevent cervical cancer. Acta Cytologica. 2020;**64**:420-424. DOI: 10.1159/000506725

[18] Venetianer R, Clarke MA, van der Marel J, Tota J, Schiffman M, Dunn ST, et al. Identification of HPV genotypes causing cervical precancer using tissue-based genotyping. International Journal of Cancer. 2020;**146**:2836-2844. DOI: 10.1002/ijc.32919

[19] Manini I, Montomoli E. Epidemiology and prevention of human papillomavirus. Annali di igiene: Medicina preventiva e di comunita. 2018;**30**:28-32. DOI: 10.7416/ai.2018.2231

[20] Chan CK, Aimagambetova G, Ukybassova T, Kongrtay K, Azizan A. Human papillomavirus infection and cervical cancer: Epidemiology, screening, and vaccination-review of current perspectives. Journal of Oncology. 2019;**2019**:3257939. DOI: 10.1155/2019/3257939

[21] Hoppe-Seyler K, Bossler F, Braun JA, Herrmann AL, Hoppe-Seyler F. The HPV E6/E7 oncogenes: Key factors for viral carcinogenesis and therapeutic targets. Trends in Microbiology. 2018;**26**:158-168. DOI: 10.1016/j.tim.2017.07.007

[22] Estevao D, Costa NR, Gil da Costa RM, Medeiros R. Hallmarks of HPV carcinogenesis: The role of E6, E7 and E5 oncoproteins in cellular malignancy. Biochim Biophys Acta Gene Regul Mech. 2019;**1862**:153-162. DOI: 10.1016/j.bbagrm.2019.01.001

[23] Gutiérrez-Hoya A, Soto-Cruz I. Role of the JAK/STAT pathway in cervical cancer: Its relationship with HPV E6/E7 oncoproteins. Cell. 2020;**9**:2297

[24] Kontomanolis EN, Koutras A, Syllaios A, Schizas D, Mastoraki A, Garmpis N, et al. Role of oncogenes and tumor-suppressor genes in carcinogenesis: A review. Anticancer Research. 2020;**40**:6009-6015. DOI: 10.21873/anticanres.14622

[25] Kontomanolis EN, Koutras A, Fasoulakis Z, Syllaios A, Diakosavvas M, Angelou K, et al. A brief overview of oncogenes and signal transduction pathways in gynecological cancer. Cancer Diagnosis & Prognosis. 2022;**2**:134-143. DOI: 10.21873/cdp.10087

[26] Oxford Textbook of Cancer Biology. Oxford, United Kingdom: Oxford University Press; 2019

[27] Chernoff J. The two-hit theory hits 50. Molecular Biology of the Cell. 2021;**32**:rt1. DOI: 10.1091/mbc.E21-08-0407

[28] Moody CA, Laimins LA. Human papillomavirus oncoproteins: Pathways to transformation. Nature Reviews. Cancer. 2010;**10**:550-560. DOI: 10.1038/nrc2886

[29] Egawa N, Egawa K, Griffin H, Doorbar J. Human papillomaviruses; epithelial tropisms, and the development of neoplasia. Viruses. 2015;7:3863-3890. DOI: 10.3390/v7072802

[30] McBride AA, Warburton A. The role of integration in oncogenic progression of HPV-associated cancers. PLoS Pathogens. 2017;**13**:e1006211. DOI: 10.1371/journal.ppat.1006211

[31] Shen-Gunther J, Cai H, Wang Y. HPV integration site mapping: A rapid method of viral integration site (VIS) analysis and visualization using automated

workflows in CLC microbial genomics. International Journal of Molecular Sciences. 2022;**23**:8132

[32] Dong G, Broker TR, Chow LT. Human papillomavirus type 11 E2 proteins repress the homologous E6 promoter by interfering with the binding of host transcription factors to adjacent elements. Journal of Virology. 1994;**68**:1115-1127. DOI: 10.1128/jvi.68.2.1115-1127.1994

[33] Tan SH, Leong LE, Walker PA, Bernard HU. The human papillomavirus type 16 E2 transcription factor binds with low cooperativity to two flanking sites and represses the E6 promoter through displacement of Sp1 and TFIID. Journal of Virology. 1994;**68**:6411-6420. DOI: 10.1128/jvi.68.10.6411-6420.1994

[34] Warburton A, Della Fera AN, McBride AA. Dangerous liaisons: Long-term replication with an extrachromosomal HPV genome. Viruses. 2021;**1846**:13

[35] Yang YK, Xi WY, Xi RX, Li JY, Li Q, Gao YE. MicroRNA-494 promotes cervical cancer proliferation through the regulation of PTEN. Oncology Reports. 2015;**33**:2393-2401. DOI: 10.3892/or.2015.3821

[36] Hanahan D. Hallmarks of cancer: New dimensions. Cancer Discovery. 2022;**12**:31-46. DOI: 10.1158/2159-8290.Cd-21-1059

[37] Morana O, Wood W, Gregory CD. The apoptosis paradox in cancer. International Journal of Molecular Sciences. 2022;**23**:1-19. DOI: 10.3390/ijms23031328

[38] Pal A, Kundu R. Human papillomavirus E6 and E7: The cervical cancer hallmarks and targets for therapy. Frontiers in Microbiology. 2019;**10**:3116. DOI: 10.3389/fmicb.2019.03116

[39] Bernard X, Robinson P, Nominé Y, Masson M, Charbonnier S, Ramirez-Ramos JR, et al. Proteasomal degradation of p53 by human papillomavirus E6 oncoprotein relies on the structural integrity of p53 core domain. PLoS One. 2011;**6**:e25981. DOI: 10.1371/journal.pone.0025981

[40] Thomas M, Banks L. Human papillomavirus (HPV) E6 interactions with Bak are conserved amongst E6 proteins from high and low risk HPV types. The Journal of General Virology. 1999;**80**(Pt 6):1513-1517. DOI: 10.1099/0022-1317-80-6-1513

[41] Filippova M, Song H, Connolly JL, Dermody TS, Duerksen-Hughes PJ. The human papillomavirus 16 E6 protein binds to tumor necrosis factor (TNF) R1 and protects cells from TNF-induced apoptosis. The Journal of Biological Chemistry. 2002;**277**:21730-21739. DOI: 10.1074/jbc.M200113200

[42] Garnett TO, Filippova M, Duerksen-Hughes PJ. Accelerated degradation of FADD and procaspase 8 in cells expressing human papilloma virus 16 E6 impairs TRAIL-mediated apoptosis. Cell Death and Differentiation. 2006;**13**:1915-1926. DOI: 10.1038/sj.cdd.4401886

[43] Aguilar-Lemarroy A, Gariglio P, Whitaker NJ, Eichhorst ST, zur Hausen H, Krammer PH, et al. Restoration of p53 expression sensitizes human papillomavirus type 16 immortalized human keratinocytes to CD95-mediated apoptosis. Oncogene. 2002;**21**:165-175. DOI: 10.1038/sj.onc.1204979

[44] Stöppler MC, Straight SW, Tsao G, Schlegel R, McCance DJ. The E5 gene of HPV-16 enhances keratinocyte immortalization by full-length DNA. Virology. 1996;**223**:251-254. DOI: 10.1006/viro.1996.0475

[45] Oh JM, Kim SH, Cho EA, Song YS, Kim WH, Juhnn YS. Human papillomavirus type 16 E5 protein inhibits hydrogen-peroxide-induced apoptosis by stimulating ubiquitin-proteasome-mediated degradation of Bax in human cervical cancer cells. Carcinogenesis. 2010;**31**:402-410. DOI: 10.1093/carcin/bgp318

[46] Kabsch K, Mossadegh N, Kohl A, Komposch G, Schenkel J, Alonso A, et al. The HPV-16 E5 protein inhibits TRAIL- and FasL-mediated apoptosis in human keratinocyte raft cultures. Intervirology. 2004;**47**:48-56. DOI: 10.1159/000076642

[47] Bailey SM. Editorial: Hallmark of cancer: Replicative immortality. Frontiers in Oncology. 2023;**13**:1204094. DOI: 10.3389/fonc.2023.1204094

[48] Souiden Y, Bouraoui A, Chaieb K, Mahdouani K. Telomeres and telomerase as targeted therapies in cancer treatment. Bulletin du Cancer. 2010;**97**:1087-1104. DOI: 10.1684/bdc.2010.1155

[49] Belgiovine C, Chiodi I, Mondello C. Telomerase: Cellular immortalization and neoplastic transformation. Multiple functions of a multifaceted complex. Cytogenetic and Genome Research. 2008;**122**:255-262. DOI: 10.1159/000167811

[50] Liu X, Dakic A, Zhang Y, Dai Y, Chen R, Schlegel R. HPV E6 protein interacts physically and functionally with the cellular telomerase complex. Proceedings of the National Academy of Sciences. 2009;**106**:18780-18785. DOI: 10.1073/pnas.0906357106

[51] Hu X, Li J, Fu M, Zhao X, Wang W. The JAK/STAT signaling pathway: From bench to clinic. Signal transduction and targeted. Therapy. 2021;**6**:402. DOI: 10.1038/s41392-021-00791-1

[52] O'Shea JJ, Schwartz DM, Villarino AV, Gadina M, McInnes IB, Laurence A. The JAK-STAT pathway: Impact on human disease and therapeutic intervention. Annual Review of Medicine. 2015;**66**:311-328. DOI: 10.1146/annurev-med-051113-024537

[53] Murray PJ. The JAK-STAT signaling pathway: Input and output integration. Journal of Immunology. 2007;**178**:2623-2629. DOI: 10.4049/jimmunol.178.5.2623

[54] Xue C, Yao Q, Gu X, Shi Q, Yuan X, Chu Q, et al. Evolving cognition of the JAK-STAT signaling pathway: Autoimmune disorders and cancer. Signal Transduction and Targeted Therapy. 2023;**8**:204. DOI: 10.1038/s41392-023-01468-7

[55] Li Q, Li Z, Luo T, Shi H. Targeting the PI3K/AKT/mTOR and RAF/MEK/ERK pathways for cancer therapy. Molecular Biomedicine. 2022;**3**:47. DOI: 10.1186/s43556-022-00110-2

[56] Steelman LS, Chappell WH, Abrams SL, Kempf RC, Long J, Laidler P, et al. Roles of the Raf/MEK/ERK and PI3K/PTEN/Akt/mTOR pathways in controlling growth and sensitivity to therapy-implications for cancer and aging. Aging (Albany NY). 2011;**3**:192-222. DOI: 10.18632/aging.100296

[57] Bossler F, Hoppe-Seyler K, Hoppe-Seyler F. PI3K/AKT/mTOR signaling regulates the virus/host cell crosstalk in HPV-positive cervical cancer cells. International Journal of Molecular Sciences. 2019;**20**:2188

[58] MacDonald BT, Tamai K, He X. Wnt/beta-catenin signaling: Components, mechanisms, and diseases. Developmental Cell. 2009;**17**:9-26. DOI: 10.1016/j.devcel.2009.06.016

[59] Stamos JL, Weis WI. The β-catenin destruction complex. Cold Spring Harbor

Perspectives in Biology. 2013;**5**:a007898. DOI: 10.1101/cshperspect.a007898

[60] Komiya Y, Habas R. Wnt signal transduction pathways. Organogenesis. 2008;**4**:68-75. DOI: 10.4161/org.4.2.5851

[61] Zhan T, Rindtorff N, Boutros M. Wnt signaling in cancer. Oncogene. 2017;**36**:1461-1473. DOI: 10.1038/onc.2016.304

[62] Liu J, Xiao Q, Xiao J, Niu C, Li Y, Zhang X, et al. Wnt/β-catenin signalling: Function, biological mechanisms, and therapeutic opportunities. Signal Transduction and Targeted Therapy. 2022;**7**:3. DOI: 10.1038/s41392-021-00762-6

[63] Zapatka M, Borozan I, Brewer DS, Iskar M, Grundhoff A, Alawi M, et al. The landscape of viral associations in human cancers. Nature Genetics. 2020;**52**:320-330. DOI: 10.1038/s41588-019-0558-9

[64] Porter VL, Marra MA. The drivers, mechanisms, and consequences of genome instability in HPV-driven cancers. Cancers. 2022;**14**:4623

[65] Parish JL, Bean AM, Park RB, Androphy EJ. ChlR1 is required for loading papillomavirus E2 onto mitotic chromosomes and viral genome maintenance. Molecular Cell. 2006;**24**:867-876. DOI: 10.1016/j.molcel.2006.11.005

[66] Sakakibara N, Mitra R, McBride AA. The papillomavirus E1 helicase activates a cellular DNA damage response in viral replication foci. Journal of Virology. 2011;**85**:8981-8995. DOI: 10.1128/jvi.00541-11

[67] Cruz-Gregorio A, Manzo-Merino J, Gonzaléz-García MC, Pedraza-Chaverri J, Medina-Campos ON, Valverde M, et al. Human papillomavirus types 16 and 18 early-expressed proteins differentially modulate the cellular redox state and DNA damage. International Journal of Biological Sciences. 2018;**14**:21-35. DOI: 10.7150/ijbs.21547

[68] Peter M, Stransky N, Couturier J, Hupé P, Barillot E, de Cremoux P, et al. Frequent genomic structural alterations at HPV insertion sites in cervical carcinoma. The Journal of Pathology. 2010;**221**:320-330. DOI: 10.1002/path.2713

[69] Halbert CL, Demers GW, Galloway DA. The E7 gene of human papillomavirus type 16 is sufficient for immortalization of human epithelial cells. Journal of Virology. 1991;**65**:473-478. DOI: 10.1128/jvi.65.1.473-478.1991

[70] Sitz J, Blanchet SA, Gameiro SF, Biquand E, Morgan TM, Galloy M, et al. Human papillomavirus E7 oncoprotein targets RNF168 to hijack the host DNA damage response. Proceedings of the National Academy of Sciences. 2019;**116**:19552-19562. DOI: 10.1073/pnas.1906102116

[71] Wallace NA, Khanal S, Robinson KL, Wendel SO, Messer JJ, Galloway DA. High-risk Alphapapillomavirus oncogenes impair the homologous recombination pathway. Journal of Virology. 2017;**91**:1-22. DOI: 10.1128/jvi.01084-01017

[72] Duensing S, Duensing A, Flores ER, Do A, Lambert PF, Münger K. Centrosome abnormalities and genomic instability by episomal expression of human papillomavirus type 16 in raft cultures of human keratinocytes. Journal of Virology. 2001;**75**:7712-7716. DOI: 10.1128/jvi.75.16.7712-7716.2001

[73] Klingelhutz AJ, Roman A. Cellular transformation by human papillomaviruses: Lessons learned by

comparing high- and low-risk viruses. Virology. 2012;**424**:77-98. DOI: 10.1016/j.virol.2011.12.018

[74] Cheung AL, Deng W. Telomere dysfunction, genome instability and cancer. Frontiers in Bioscience. 2008;**13**:2075-2090. DOI: 10.2741/2825

[75] Widschwendter A, Müller HM, Hubalek MM, Wiedemair A, Fiegl H, Goebel G, et al. Methylation status and expression of human telomerase reverse transcriptase in ovarian and cervical cancer. Gynecologic Oncology. 2004;**93**:407-416. DOI: 10.1016/j.ygyno.2004.01.036

[76] Warburg O. On the origin of cancer cells. Science. 1956;**123**:309-314. DOI: 10.1126/science.123.3191.309

[77] Vinay Kumar AKA, Aster JC. Robbins Basic Pathology. 10th ed. Philadelphia, USA: Elsevier—Health Sciences Division; 2023

[78] Bast RC, Kufe DW, Pollock RE, Weichselbaum RR, Holland JF, Frei E. Holland-Frei Cancer Medicine. 10th ed. Hoboken, New Jersey: John Wiley and Sons; 2023

[79] Kennelly PJ, Botham KM, McGuinness OP, Rodwell VW, Weil P. Harper's Illustrated Biochemistry. 32nd ed. New York: McGraw Hill; 2023

[80] Yuan Y, Cai X, Shen F, Ma F. HPV post-infection microenvironment and cervical cancer. Cancer Letters. 2021;**497**:243-254. DOI: 10.1016/j.canlet.2020.10.034

[81] Brand KA, Hermfisse U. Aerobic glycolysis by proliferating cells: A protective strategy against reactive oxygen species1. The FASEB Journal. 1997;**11**:388-395. DOI: 10.1096/fasebj.11.5.9141507

[82] Torresano L, Nuevo-Tapioles C, Santacatterina F, Cuezva JM. Metabolic reprogramming and disease progression in cancer patients. Biochimica et Biophysica Acta (BBA)—Molecular Basis of Disease. 1866;**2020**:165721. DOI: 10.1016/j.bbadis.2020.165721

[83] Ilhan ZE, Łaniewski P, Thomas N, Roe DJ, Chase DM, Herbst-Kralovetz MM. Deciphering the complex interplay between microbiota, HPV, inflammation and cancer through cervicovaginal metabolic profiling. eBioMedicine. 2019;**44**:675-690. DOI: 10.1016/j.ebiom.2019.04.028

[84] Zhang R, Su J, Xue SL, Yang H, Ju LL, Ji Y, et al. HPV E6/p53 mediated down-regulation of miR-34a inhibits Warburg effect through targeting LDHA in cervical cancer. American Journal of Cancer Research. 2016;**6**:312-320

[85] Henke E, Nandigama R, Ergün S. Extracellular matrix in the tumor microenvironment and its impact on cancer therapy. Frontiers in Molecular Biosciences. 2019;**6**:160. DOI: 10.3389/fmolb.2019.00160

[86] Anderson NM, Simon MC. The tumor microenvironment. Current Biology. 2020;**30**:R921-R925. DOI: 10.1016/j.cub.2020.06.081

[87] Hanahan D, Coussens LM. Accessories to the crime: Functions of cells recruited to the tumor microenvironment. Cancer Cell. 2012;**21**:309-322. DOI: 10.1016/j.ccr.2012.02.022

[88] Balkwill FR, Capasso M, Hagemann T. The tumor microenvironment at a glance. Journal of Cell Science. 2012;**125**:5591-5596. DOI: 10.1242/jcs.116392

[89] Cisneros-Villanueva M, Hidalgo-Pérez L, Rios-Romero M,

Cedro-Tanda A, Ruiz-Villavicencio CA, Page K, et al. Cell-free DNA analysis in current cancer clinical trials: A review. British Journal of Cancer. 2022;**126**:391-400. DOI: 10.1038/s41416-021-01696-0

[90] Lin D, Shen L, Luo M, Zhang K, Li J, Yang Q, et al. Circulating tumor cells: Biology and clinical significance. Signal Transduction and Targeted Therapy. 2021;**6**:404. DOI: 10.1038/s41392-021-00817-8

[91] Li I, Nabet BY. Exosomes in the tumor microenvironment as mediators of cancer therapy resistance. Molecular Cancer. 2019;**18**:32. DOI: 10.1186/s12943-019-0975-5

[92] Monteran L, Erez N. The dark side of fibroblasts: Cancer-associated fibroblasts as mediators of immunosuppression in the tumor microenvironment. Frontiers in Immunology. 1835;**2019**:10. DOI: 10.3389/fimmu.2019.01835

[93] Lisanti MP, Martinez-Outschoorn UE, Chiavarina B, Pavlides S, Whitaker-Menezes D, Tsirigos A, et al. Understanding the "lethal" drivers of tumor-stroma co-evolution. Cancer Biology & Therapy. 2010;**10**:537-542. DOI: 10.4161/cbt.10.6.13370

[94] Tang Y, Zhang AXJ, Chen G, Wu Y, Gu W. Prognostic and therapeutic TILs of cervical cancer—Current advances and future perspectives. Molecular Therapy - Oncolytics. 2021;**22**:410-430. DOI: 10.1016/j.omto.2021.07.006

[95] Ma W, Wang K, Du J, Luan J, Lou G. Multi-dose parecoxib provides an immunoprotective effect by balancing T helper 1 (Th1), Th2, Th17 and regulatory T cytokines following laparoscopy in patients with cervical cancer. Molecular Medicine Reports. 2015;**11**:2999-3008. DOI: 10.3892/mmr.2014.3003

[96] Lin W, Niu Z, Zhang H, Kong Y, Wang Z, Yang X, et al. Imbalance of Th1/Th2 and Th17/Treg during the development of uterine cervical cancer. International Journal of Clinical and Experimental Pathology. 2019;**12**:3604-3612

[97] Balkwill F. Cancer and the chemokine network. Nature Reviews. Cancer. 2004;**4**:540-550. DOI: 10.1038/nrc1388

[98] Wang S, Liu R, Yu Q, Dong L, Bi Y, Liu G. Metabolic reprogramming of macrophages during infections and cancer. Cancer Letters. 2019;**452**:14-22. DOI: 10.1016/j.canlet.2019.03.015

[99] Petrillo M, Zannoni GF, Martinelli E, Pedone Anchora L, Ferrandina G, Tropeano G, et al. Polarisation of tumor-associated macrophages toward M2 phenotype correlates with poor response to chemoradiation and reduced survival in patients with locally advanced cervical Cancer. PLoS One. 2015;**10**:e0136654. DOI: 10.1371/journal.pone.0136654

[100] Hillen F, Griffioen AW. Tumour vascularization: Sprouting angiogenesis and beyond. Cancer Metastasis Reviews. 2007;**26**:489-502. DOI: 10.1007/s10555-007-9094-7

[101] Folkman J, D'Amore PA. Blood vessel formation: What is its molecular basis? Cell. 1996;**87**:1153-1155. DOI: 10.1016/S0092-8674(00)81810-3

[102] Albrecht ED, Babischkin JS, Lidor Y, Anderson LD, Udoff LC, Pepe GJ. Effect of estrogen on angiogenesis in co-cultures of human endometrial cells and microvascular endothelial cells. Human Reproduction. 2003;**18**:2039-2047. DOI: 10.1093/humrep/deg415

[103] Appelmann I, Liersch R, Kessler T, Mesters RM, Berdel WE. Angiogenesis

inhibition in cancer therapy: Platelet-derived growth factor (PDGF) and vascular endothelial growth factor (VEGF) and their receptors: Biological functions and role in malignancy. Recent Results in Cancer Research. 2010;**180**:51-81. DOI: 10.1007/978-3-540-78281-0_5

[104] Martínez CE, Smith PC, Palma Alvarado VA. The influence of platelet-derived products on angiogenesis and tissue repair: A concise update. Frontiers in Physiology. 2015;**6**:1-7. DOI: 10.3389/fphys.2015.00290

[105] Bergers G, Benjamin LE. Tumorigenesis and the angiogenic switch. Nature Reviews Cancer. 2003;**3**:401-410. DOI: 10.1038/nrc1093

[106] Wu MP, Tzeng CC, Wu LW, Huang KF, Chou CY. Thrombospondin-1 acts as a fence to inhibit angiogenesis that occurs during cervical carcinogenesis. Cancer Journal. 2004;**10**:27-32. DOI: 10.1097/00130404-200401000-00007

[107] Baeriswyl V, Christofori G. The angiogenic switch in carcinogenesis. Seminars in Cancer Biology. 2009;**19**:329-337. DOI: 10.1016/j.semcancer.2009.05.003

[108] Rofstad EK, Sundfør K, Lyng H, Tropé CG. Hypoxia-induced treatment failure in advanced squamous cell carcinoma of the uterine cervix is primarily due to hypoxia-induced radiation resistance rather than hypoxia-induced metastasis. British Journal of Cancer. 2000;**83**:354-359. DOI: 10.1054/bjoc.2000.1266

[109] Brown LM, Cowen RL, Debray C, Eustace A, Erler JT, Sheppard FC, et al. Reversing hypoxic cell chemoresistance in vitro using genetic and small molecule approaches targeting hypoxia inducible factor-1. Molecular Pharmacology. 2006;**69**:411-418. DOI: 10.1124/mol.105.015743

[110] Du R, Lu KV, Petritsch C, Liu P, Ganss R, Passegué E, et al. HIF1alpha induces the recruitment of bone marrow-derived vascular modulatory cells to regulate tumor angiogenesis and invasion. Cancer Cell. 2008;**13**:206-220. DOI: 10.1016/j.ccr.2008.01.034

[111] Ferrara N. VEGF and the quest for tumour angiogenesis factors. Nature Reviews. Cancer. 2002;**2**:795-803. DOI: 10.1038/nrc909

[112] Goodsell DS. The molecular perspective: VEGF and angiogenesis. Stem Cells. 2003;**21**:118-119. DOI: 10.1634/stemcells.21-1-118

[113] Pepper MS, Ferrara N, Orci L, Montesano R. Potent synergism between vascular endothelial growth factor and basic fibroblast growth factor in the induction of angiogenesis in vitro. Biochemical and Biophysical Research Communications. 1992;**189**:824-831. DOI: 10.1016/0006-291x(92)92277-5

[114] Giavazzi R, Sennino B, Coltrini D, Garofalo A, Dossi R, Ronca R, et al. Distinct role of fibroblast growth factor-2 and vascular endothelial growth factor on tumor growth and angiogenesis. The American Journal of Pathology. 2003;**162**:1913-1926. DOI: 10.1016/s0002-9440(10)64325-8

[115] Fujii T, Kuwano H. Regulation of the expression balance of angiopoietin-1 and angiopoietin-2 by Shh and FGF-2. In Vitro Cellular & Developmental Biology. Animal. 2010;**46**:487-491. DOI: 10.1007/s11626-009-9270-x

[116] Nasarre P, Thomas M, Kruse K, Helfrich I, Wolter V, Deppermann C, et al. Host-derived angiopoietin-2 affects early stages of tumor development and

vessel maturation but is dispensable for later stages of tumor growth. Cancer Research. 2009;**69**:1324-1333. DOI: 10.1158/0008-5472.Can-08-3030

[117] Monk BJ, Sill MW, Burger RA, Gray HJ, Buekers TE, Roman LD. Phase II trial of bevacizumab in the treatment of persistent or recurrent squamous cell carcinoma of the cervix: A gynecologic oncology group study. Journal of Clinical Oncology. 2009;**27**:1069-1074. DOI: 10.1200/jco.2008.18.9043

[118] Ikeda Y, Takano M, Oda K, Kouta H, Goto T, Kudoh K, et al. Weekly administration of bevacizumab, gemcitabine, and oxaliplatin in patients with recurrent and refractory ovarian cancer: A preliminary result of 19 cases. International Journal of Gynecological Cancer. 2013;**23**:355-360. DOI: 10.1097/IGC.0b013e31827de69e

[119] Schefter TE, Winter K, Kwon JS, Stuhr K, Balaraj K, Yaremko BP, et al. A phase II study of bevacizumab in combination with definitive radiotherapy and cisplatin chemotherapy in untreated patients with locally advanced cervical carcinoma: Preliminary results of RTOG 0417. International Journal of Radiation Oncology, Biology, Physics. 2012;**83**:1179-1184. DOI: 10.1016/j.ijrobp.2011.10.060

[120] Schefter T, Winter K, Kwon JS, Stuhr K, Balaraj K, Yaremko BP, et al. RTOG 0417: Efficacy of bevacizumab in combination with definitive radiation therapy and cisplatin chemotherapy in untreated patients with locally advanced cervical carcinoma. International Journal of Radiation Oncology, Biology, Physics. 2014;**88**:101-105. DOI: 10.1016/j.ijrobp.2013.10.022

[121] Liu P, Zhang C, Liao Y, Liu J, Huang J, Xia M, et al. High expression of PTPRM predicts poor prognosis and promotes tumor growth and lymph node metastasis in cervical cancer. Cell Death & Disease. 2020;**11**:687. DOI: 10.1038/s41419-020-02826-x

[122] Cui J, Zhang C, Lee J-E, Bartholdy BA, Yang D, Liu Y, et al. MLL3 loss drives metastasis by promoting a hybrid epithelial–mesenchymal transition state. Nature Cell Biology. 2023;**25**:145-158. DOI: 10.1038/s41556-022-01045-0

[123] Vasaikar SV, Deshmukh AP, den Hollander P, Addanki S, Kuburich NA, Kudaravalli S, et al. EMTome: A resource for pan-cancer analysis of epithelial-mesenchymal transition genes and signatures. British Journal of Cancer. 2021;**124**:259-269. DOI: 10.1038/s41416-020-01178-9

[124] Yang J, Antin P, Berx G, Blanpain C, Brabletz T, Bronner M, et al. Guidelines and definitions for research on epithelial–mesenchymal transition. Nature Reviews Molecular Cell Biology. 2020;**21**:341-352. DOI: 10.1038/s41580-020-0237-9

[125] Vergara D, Simeone P, Franck J, Trerotola M, Giudetti A, Capobianco L, et al. Translating epithelial mesenchymal transition markers into the clinic: Novel insights from proteomics. EuPA Open Proteomics. 2016;**10**:31-41. DOI: 10.1016/j.euprot.2016.01.003

[126] Konieczny P, Adamus T, Sułkowski M, Skrzypek K, Majka M. Impact of AMPK on cervical carcinoma progression and metastasis. Cell Death & Disease. 2023;**14**:43. DOI: 10.1038/s41419-023-05583-9

Chapter 2

Radiotherapy in Cervical Cancer

Shraddha Srivastava, Nara Singh Moirangthem, Arunima Ghosh, Indrajeet Gupta and Madan Lal Brahma Bhatt

Abstract

Radiotherapy plays a significant role in the management of cervix cancer. In recent decades, there have been several advancements in radiation therapy treatment techniques. Moving from conventional two-dimensional techniques to advanced techniques like 3D conformal radiation therapy (3D-CRT), intensity-modulated radiation therapy (IMRT), and volumetric modulated radiation therapy (VMAT) has led to improvement in the treatment outcomes. The aim of radiation therapy is achieved by these advanced techniques, which deliver optimal tumoricidal doses to tumor volumes and minimal doses to the normal tissues around the tumor and can reduce toxicity more effectively than the conventional techniques. These external beam radiotherapy (EBRT) techniques along with brachytherapy play a significant role in the treatment of gynaecological cancer. Compared to point-based dose brachytherapy planning, better local control and lower toxicity have been associated with advanced image-based brachytherapy.

Keywords: radiotherapy, 3DCRT, IMRT, cervical cancer, brachytherapy

1. Introduction

Cervical carcinoma is the fourth most common malignancy in women worldwide [1]. According to GLOBOCAN 2020 statistics, estimated new cases of cervix cancer worldwide are 604,127 (3.1%) estimated deaths are 341,831 (3.4%). In India, the incidence of cervix cancer is 123,907 (9.4%), while mortality in such cases is 77,348 (9.1%) [2]. Cervical cancer cases are predominant in Asia, Africa, and Central and South America due to lesser frequency of screening, multiparity, low-socioeconomic status, poor hygiene, low immunity and nutritional problems [3]. Most cases are in Africa because of fewer screening measures and the chances of immunodeficiency because of the human immunodeficiency virus (HIV). More than 90% of cervical cancers are related to human papillomavirus (HPV) infection and are sexually transmitted [4]. Intrauterine exposure to diethylstilbestrol (DES) is related to the development of adenocarcinoma.

Radiotherapy plays a significant role in the management of cervix cancer. The standard mode of definitive treatment in patients of locally advanced cervical carcinoma involves both components of radiotherapy: External beam radiotherapy (EBRT) and brachytherapy [5, 6].

2. Rationale for the use of radiotherapy in cervical cancer

To achieve excellent locoregional control (LRC), disease-free survival (DFS) and overall survival (OS), surgery or radiotherapy alone is recommended for FIGO stage I, with tumor size less than 4 cm. Radiotherapy alone has also helped to achieve excellent survival and pelvic disease control rates in patients with stage IB cervical cancer. Eifel et al. reported 5-year disease-specific survival and pelvic control rates of 90 and 98%, respectively, for 701 patients treated with radiation alone for stage IB1 disease [7].

Concurrent chemoradiotherapy (CCRT) is the standard treatment of choice for locally advanced cervical cancer (LACC) ((FIGO (International Federation of Gynecology and Obstetrics) stage IIB to IVA). The survival outcome with CCRT is better when compared to radiotherapy alone [8–11].

3. External beam therapy

3.1 Indications and target volumes

External beam therapy (EBRT) is part of the routine treatment of Carcinoma Cervix FIGO stages IB2 to IVA and in some earlier stages if the patient is not fit for/willing for surgical treatment [12, 13]. In patients with an intact uterus, EBRT is planned to treat the primary tumour with its local extensions as determined by clinical examination and diagnostic imaging, i.e. Gross tumour Volume (GTV), along with the entire uterus, the cervix, 2–3 cm of vagina below the inferior most extent of the disease, the parametrium and uterosacral ligaments. This forms the Primary-Clinical Target Volume (CTV – P). EBRT also targets the draining lymph nodal groups, i.e. the pelvic group of lymph nodes, which includes the internal, external, common iliac nodes, obturator and presacral lymph nodes. This forms the Nodal—Clinical Target Volume (CTV – N). In certain cases, the para-aortic or inguinal group of lymph nodes may also be treated by EBRT [14–16].

Para-aortic group of lymph nodes may be treated electively in cases where multiple pelvic nodes are involved (i.e. > 2 pathological LN or involvement of common iliac region). Therapeutic para-aortic irradiation is done in FIGO stage IIIC2 patients. In patients where the lower one-third of the vagina is involved, i.e. FIGO stage IIIA, the inguinal group of nodes must also be treated electively [13].

When EBRT is administered in patients post-hysterectomy, the radiation field includes the CTV-P, which comprises the tumor bed and any possible uterosacral, parametrial, uterine extension, and the CTV-N. Indications of adjuvant EBRT could be the presence of intermediate-or high-risk pathological features such as lymphovascular space involvement or stromal invasion, the large size of the tumor, involvement of lymph nodes or parametria and gross/microscopic residual disease post-surgery [9, 17].

3.2 EBRT treatment techniques

3.2.1 Two-dimensional conventional radiotherapy technique

Conventionally, EBRT is planned and administered based on bony anatomy as seen on X-ray simulation and as per clinical judgment of tumour location and extension, i.e. 2-D treatment planning.

Since there is limited soft tissue contrast seen on radiographs, treatment planning is done based on knowledge of tumor position relative to bony landmarks and anatomical structures visible with the aid of contrast agents such as barium which may be used to visualize small bowel or lower extent of disease in the vagina. For the treatment of gynecological malignancies, patients are generally simulated in the supine position as it is easily reproducible and more comfortable for the patient. A prone position may also be used for obese patients to reduce radiation dose to the bowel. It is important to ensure that patients are simulated and treated daily with a full bladder to reduce bowel toxicity.

When anteroposterior (AP) patient thickness is <20 cm, patients are treated by two fields (AP-PA) (**Figure 1(a)** and **(b)**), and when AP thickness is >20 cm, patients are treated by four fields (AP-PA and bilateral, i.e. box field technique) (**Figure 2(a)** and **(b)**). **Figures 1(b)** and **2(b)** represent Beam's eye view for AP and AP-lateral field respectively. Box field technique is to be strongly considered for AP thickness > 20 cm and treatment on Cobalt teletherapy units. For conventional whole pelvic radiotherapy (WPRT), the superior border of the field is placed at L4-L5 interspace while the inferior border of the field is at the lower border of the obturator foramen or 2–3 cm below the vaginal extent of disease, whichever is lower. The lateral borders of the AP/PA field extend 1.5–2 cm lateral from the widest point of the pelvic brim. The lateral fields cover the sacral hollow posteriorly, extending 0.5–1 cm anterior to the pubic symphysis. Shielding blocks may be placed at the corners of the field to reduce the dose to the small bowel, femoral heads and sacrum.

For para-aortic field irradiation, the pelvic field may be extended superiorly uptoT12-L1 interspace, in continuation with the pelvic field, or a separate para-aortic field may be set up with a gap from the superior border of the pelvic field to maintain dose homogeneity. Four fields technique (including AP-PA and two lateral fields) are used to treat para-aortic nodal involvement to reduce small bowel dose. When the inguinal group of lymph nodes is to be irradiated, the lateral extent of the AP/PA fields is extended up to the greater trochanter. When indicated, a parametrial boost dose may be administered after making a midline shielding block, although this technique is largely being replaced by interstitial brachytherapy [18].

Even though modern guidelines recommend the use of CT/MRI/PET-based planning, due to resource constraints, several treatment centres in Low-Middle-Income Countries (LMIC) still use 2-D treatment planning.

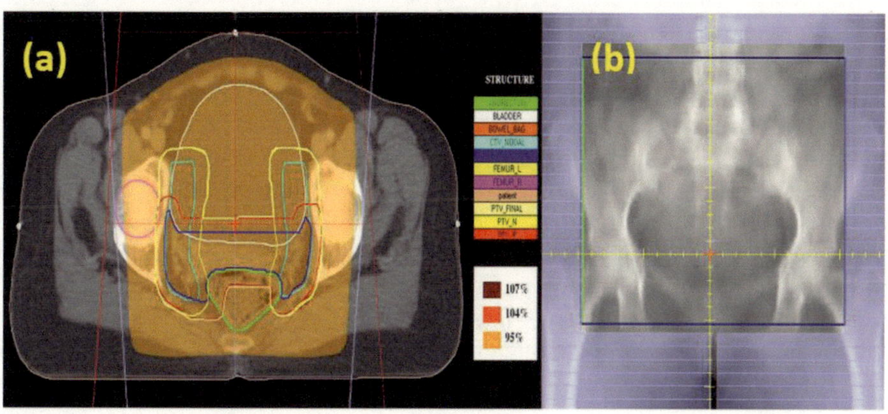

Figure 1.
(a) Two field conventional AP-PA plan, (b) Beam's eye view-AP field.

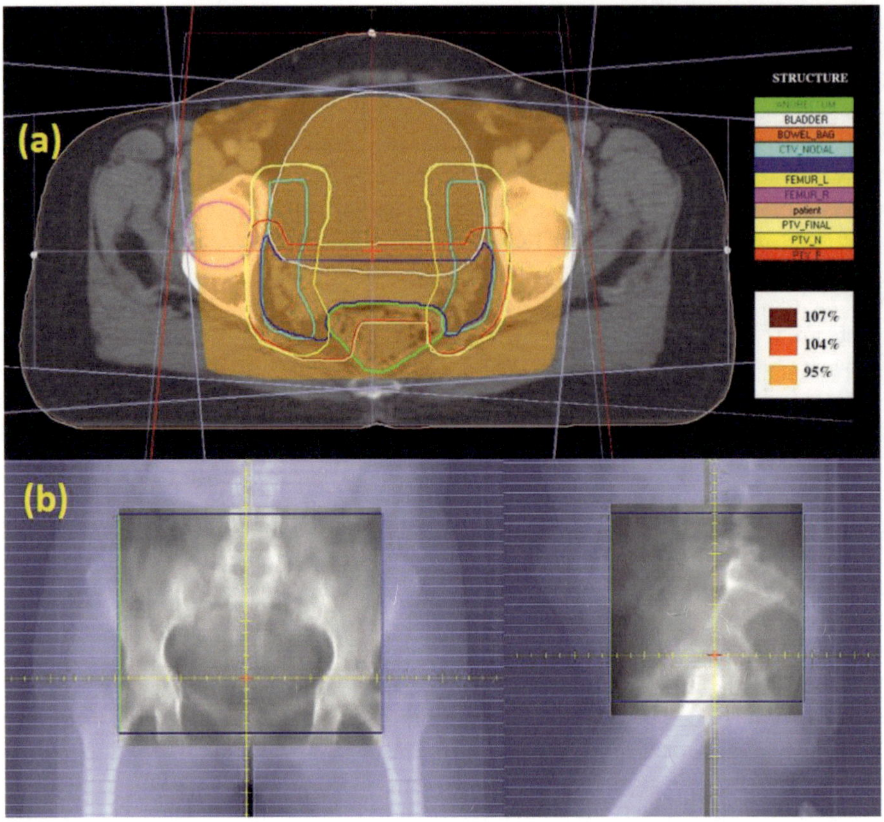

Figure 2.
(a) Four field conventional box-field plan (b) Beam's eye view-AP and lateral.

3.2.2 Three-dimensional conformal radiotherapy

Several studies have shown that planning on CT/MRI gives better coverage of CTV-N and CTV-P as compared to 2-D treatment planning, where geographical blunders can quickly happen, especially for CTV-N. Thus, CT-based planning (along with the incorporation of MRI/PET when available, preferably taken with the patient in treatment position) has now become the standard for EBRT in cervical cancer treatment planning in most developed countries.

For 3D-Conformal Radiotherapy (3D-CRT), the patient is simulated after administration of intravenous contrast as the vasculatures serve as a surrogate for the delineation of CTV-N. At the time of CT simulation, radio-opaque markers are placed for identification of the vaginal extent of disease and at the introitus of the vagina and anal verge to help delineate normal structures. Patient position during simulation is as explained earlier. Administration of oral contrast 30 minutes before simulation may help in better delineation of the small bowel. The CTV-P, CTV-N and organs at risk (OARs) are contoured on the axial CT sections acquired at the time of simulation as per standard guidelines and the clinician's judgment. Superiorly, the CTV-N extends from the bifurcation of the common iliac vessels as visualized on the CT scans, which may lie at a higher vertebral level compared to the conventionally placed superior border of the 2D technique. Inferiorly, CTV-N extends to cover the external iliac, internal iliac, presacral and obturator groups of lymph nodes. Planning target volumes (PTVs)

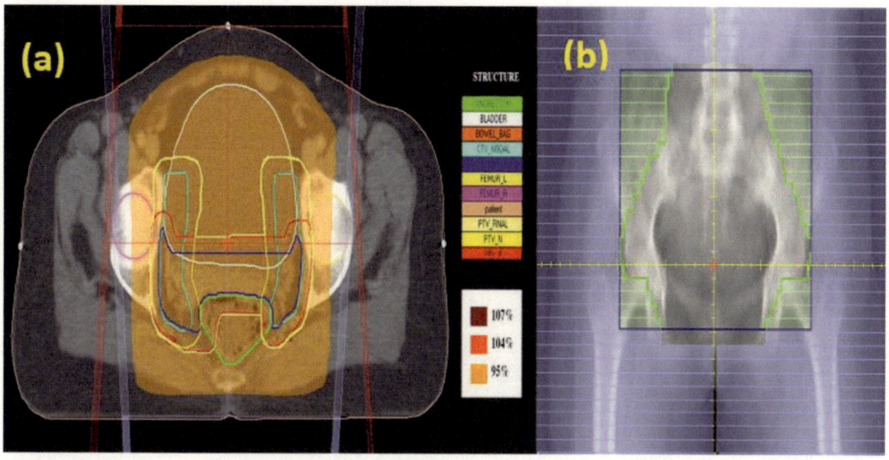

Figure 3.
(a) Two field AP-PA 3D-CRT plan (b) DRR- AP field.

are created for each CTV (CTV-P and CTV-N) as per institutional standards. The common organs at risks (OARs) used in treatment planning are the bowel, bladder, rectum and femoral heads.

Similar to the 2D treatment technique, the patient can be treated with two fields (AP-PA) (**Figure 3(a)** and **(b)**) or box fields (**Figure 4(a)** and **(b)**), arrangement of beams of 6 and/or 15 MV depending on the patient's AP thickness and disease. When indicated, para-aortic/parametrial boost volumes may also be included in the planning volumes [18]. **Figures 3(b)** and **4(b)** represent digitally reconstructed radiographs (DRR) of AP and AP-Lateral field respectively.

Moderns LNACs are equipped with multileaf collimators (MLCs), which are small, individually motorized leaves that can be used to shape the treatment field and block normal tissues such as skin, soft muscle tissue, anterior small bowel, parts of anorectum to reduce normal tissue toxicity as compared to 2D treatment planning [18, 19].

3.2.3 Intensity-modulated radiation treatment

2D and 3D radiation techniques have several limitations, such as encompassing large volumes of normal tissues in the treatment fields, which leads to several acute and long-term complications such as gastrointestinal, hematological and genitourinary complications and also the difficulty to deliver higher doses higher and potentially more efficacious doses to select patients at increased risk of recurrence, for example, those with involved lymph nodes and gross unresectable disease [20, 21].

The use of Intensity Modulated Radiation Therapy (IMRT)/Volumetric Modulated Arc Therapy (VMAT) is now being recommended by international guidelines for EBRT for cervical cancer as several studies have shown reduced treatment-related toxicities and improved survival for patients treated with these treatment techniques. With the aid of IMRT, it is possible to deliver complex dose distributions for target volumes and facilitate rapid dose fall-off outside the target volume. Unlike the convex-shaped dose distribution given by a 3D-CRT plan, an IMRT plan involves the superposition of multiple-segmented fields from different directions, which results in a dose distribution that is concave in shape around the OARs when PTVs are in close proximity to them thus aiding in reducing the dose delivered to the former [22].

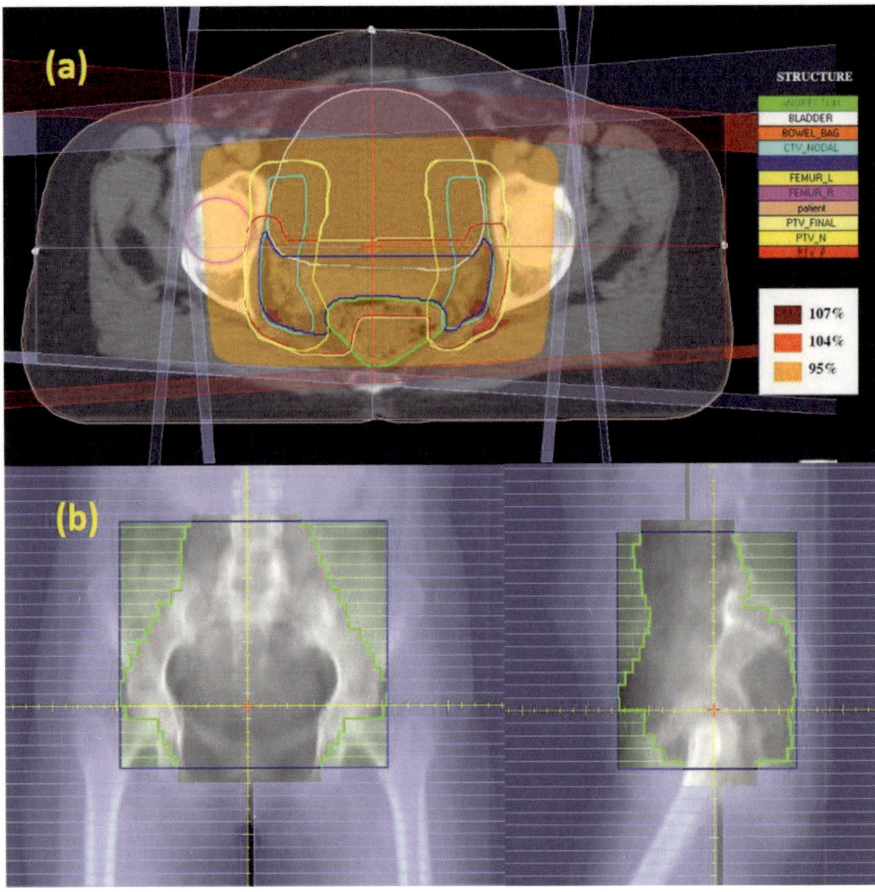

Figure 4.
(a) Four field 3D-CRT plan (b) DRR- AP and lateral field.

When patients with intact uterus are planned for IMRT treatment, patients are simulated with a full bladder as well as an empty bladder, and both the CT simulations films are fused to estimate internal target volume (ITV) margins. Custom immobilization devices such as body mold that fixes the position of the upper body, trunk and proximal legs are recommended to reduce set-up error. After CT simulations and contouring of target volumes and organs at risk on axial sections, multiple (5–7) non-coplanar treatment beams are placed for the IMRT process, which could be placed manually by treatment planners or could be automatically shown in **Figure 5**. The next steps in IMRT treatment planning involve determining the plan objectives, i.e. target dose and coverage and normal tissue doses, followed by optimization of intensity distribution, dose calculation by inverse planning and treatment plan evaluation. MLCs shape or modulate the intensity of the treatment field and help in the delivery of IMRT while improving the therapeutic ratio [19].

3.3 Image-guided radiotherapy

Image-guided Radiotherapy (IGRT) is recommended along with IMRT/VMAT to limit PTV margins and ensure safe dose delivery. IGRT is important for target

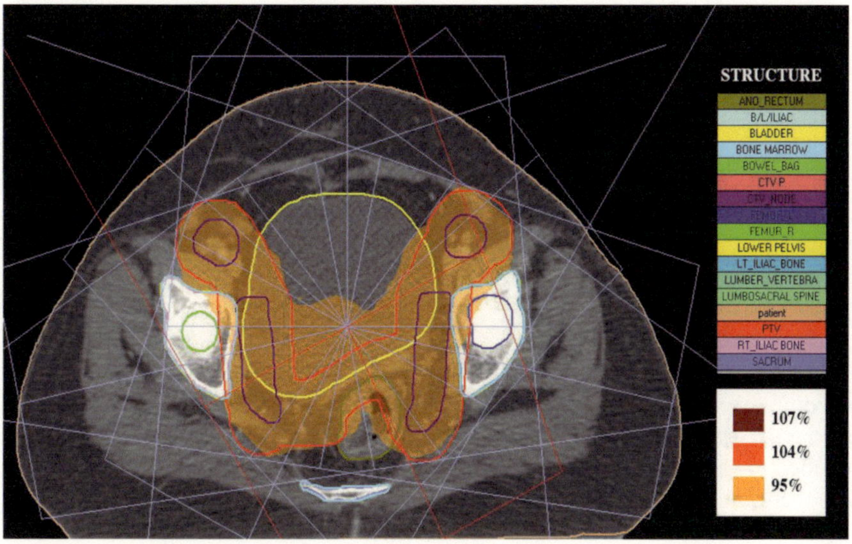

Figure 5.
IMRT of cervix cancer with beam arrangement.

delineation as well as for treatment delivery. The most commonly used IGRT treatment delivery technology is electronic portal devices (EPIDs), followed by kilovoltage (kV) and megavoltage (MV) CBCT and helical tomotherapy. IMRT/VMAT can also be used to safely deliver boost doses to pathological pelvic or para-aortic lymph nodes safely as compared to 3D-CRT. IMRT-SIB can be used in such patients, i.e. FIGO stage IIIC to deliver adequate doses without increasing overall treatment times (OTT). EBRT delivered by IG-IMRT in adjuvant settings has reduced toxicity with no difference in disease outcomes. Although IMRT is not considered an alternative to brachytherapy, in certain patients where brachytherapy is not an option due to the extensive nature of the disease, IMRT/SBRT boosts have been used as a last resort [23, 24].

3.4 Radiation dose and treatment schedule

Patients are treated by EBRT to a dose of 45Gy/25 fractions or 46Gy/23 fractions [13]. An additional boost dose of up to 60 Gy can be delivered to grossly involved nodes. A parametrial boost of 5–10 Gy may be given to bulky parametrium/pelvic sidewall disease after completion of WPRT [13, 25].

When treating with curative intent, EBRT should include concurrent cisplatin-based chemotherapy administration, as several trials and meta-analyses have shown benefits in locoregional control as well as overall survival [26]. EBRT is followed by brachytherapy for optimal tumor control.

3.5 Role of EBRT in salvage and palliative

In patients with locoregional recurrent disease, CTRT can be offered to radiotherapy naïve patients. EBRT can be combined with brachytherapy in pelvic centrally recurrent disease.

Palliative EBRT may be given to patients with painful local disease, symptomatic bone metastases or vaginal bleeding [13].

4. Brachytherapy

Brachytherapy is a technique to deliver radiation at a short distance using an encapsulated source. The sources are placed close to or into the treatment volume. It can be delivered in different ways. The most common technique used in the treatment of cervical cancer is intracavitary brachytherapy. In cases where intracavitary brachytherapy is not feasible, interstitial brachytherapy is used for the treatment. These techniques have been discussed below.

4.1 History of brachytherapy

In the beginning, radium was the only radionuclide used for intracavitary treatment, which was later discontinued due to reasons concerning radiation safety. It was replaced with other radionuclides like Cs-137, Ir-192 and Co-60. Ir-192 and Co-60 are the most popular gamma-emitting source used in ICBT. Initially, manual after-loading techniques were used for the treatment, which caused radiation exposure to the personnel involved in the procedure, but with the introduction of remote after-loading units, the personnel exposure was eliminated. These machines have a mechanism to move and retract the source automatically. The source moves in steps and irradiates each position for a planned dwell time. The dose rate has been a crucial parameter in determining the impact of radiation on target and normal structures.

Low-dose rate brachytherapy machines with Cs-137 sources have been used for the treatment of cervix cancer for decades. However, they have gradually been phased out due to high patient bulk and lengthy treatment duration. The use of high dose rate (HDR) machines for intracavitary brachytherapy treatment has increased due to several advantages like shorter treatment time, increased patient treatment, etc. Due to these profound differences, HDR machines have become predominant worldwide.

In earlier times, when treatment planning was not based on computers and computation of absorbed dose was limited, to determine the number of sources, their arrangement, strength and the dose distribution, it was necessary to define some rules. Therefore, different dosimetric systems were developed for brachytherapy. Stockholm system in 1914, the Paris system (1919) and the Manchester system in (1938) were the systems used for intracavitary brachytherapy [27]. However, Stockholm and Paris systems did not gain popularity as they were based on the description of absorbed dose based on mg-hrs of radium used and did not assess absorbed dose well in tumors and organs at risk. Manchester system came to be used worldwide as it involved clear specification of absorbed dose at point A and to critical structures.

With the introduction of the Manchester system, the concept of absorbed dose point prescription came into existence. The purpose of dose points was to obtain a method of dose prescribing and reporting which was reproducible on orthogonal radiographs in terms of anatomy or applicator. Taking this into consideration, Point A was defined by Tod and Meredith in 1938, and was later modified in 1953 [28]. They defined it as a point located 2 cm superior to the last intrauterine source and 2 cm lateral to the cervical canal. Manchester system also considered Point B, which represented the dose to internal iliac and obturator lymph nodes. Since the bladder and rectum were the critical structures that were most affected during ICBT of cervix cancer, it was necessary to record the doses received by them. Therefore, besides the point A dose, the dose to bladder and rectum points, pelvic wall point [29] and lymphatic trapezoid [30] were also estimated. The doses to points representing the bladder and rectum were recommended to be below 80% of the dose prescribed to Point A.

4.2 Treatment techniques

4.2.1 Intracavitary brachytherapy (ICBT)

Intracavitary brachytherapy (ICBT) is a technique where sources are placed in body cavities [31]. It has been widely used in the treatment of gynecological malignancies [32]. The technique employs specific applicators inserted in the uterus and vagina to deliver high-dose radiotherapy [33] by creating a volumetric dose distribution around the tumor. It has an important role in the management of cervical cancer. ICBT can be used either solely for treatment in the early stages or in combination with EBRT (locally advanced cases). Since a very high dose to the primary cervical tumor and a relatively lower dose to the nearby critical structures can be delivered by ICBT, better local control and less toxicity can be achieved using intracavitary brachytherapy [34–36]. In fact, a decline in survival rates has been observed in patients where brachytherapy after EBRT is not given [37, 38]. Therefore, ICBT becomes a necessary part of the whole treatment regime. Ir-192 is the most common source used for HDR brachytherapy in cervical cancer. However, recently, Co-60-based HDR brachytherapy has gained popularity for ICRT in cervix cancer as it reduces the cost of frequent source replacement due to its longer half-life [39].

4.2.2 Interstitial brachytherapy

It is a method where radioactive sources are implanted directly into the tumor tissue. This technique can be used in sites where head and neck, prostate and soft tissue sarcoma. In cervical carcinoma cases where intracavitary technique is not feasible due to various factors such as involvement of medial parametrium, bulky tumor (size >4 cm) and recurrent disease, interstitial brachytherapy is a preferred technique [40]. Interstitial implants use trans-perineal [41] or trans-vaginal templates [42]. Martinez Universal Perineal Interstitial Template (MUPIT) is one such template designed to deliver brachytherapy doses [43]. Dose prescription points in interstitial brachytherapy are defined using the rules of Paris system.

4.3 Image-based brachytherapy

4.3.1 Two-dimensional image-based brachytherapy

Initially, applicators used in the Manchester system consisted of two ovoids, an intrauterine tube (made of rubber), and a low-dose-rate brachytherapy machine were used for treatment. However, with the evolution in technology, the HDR machines and modern applicators like Fletcher Williamson stainless steel applicators consisting of two ovoids (diameter 20, 25 and 30 mm) and a uterine tandem (angles 15°, 30° and 45°) came into existence (**Figure 6**).

In the ICRT technique, the tandem is inserted in the uterine canal, and ovoids are placed in vaginal fornices in OT. After the completion of the application, treatment planning of patients is done on anterior-posterior and lateral orthogonal x-ray images in the treatment planning system (TPS). This involves reconstruction of the applicator, loading the source positions and calculation of the doses to Point A, ICRU bladder point and ICRU rectal points. Reporting doses to ICRU bladder and ICRU rectal points are recommended by ICRU report 38 [44]. The ICRU bladder point is identified with the help of a contrast-filled Foley's bulb. While ICRU rectal point

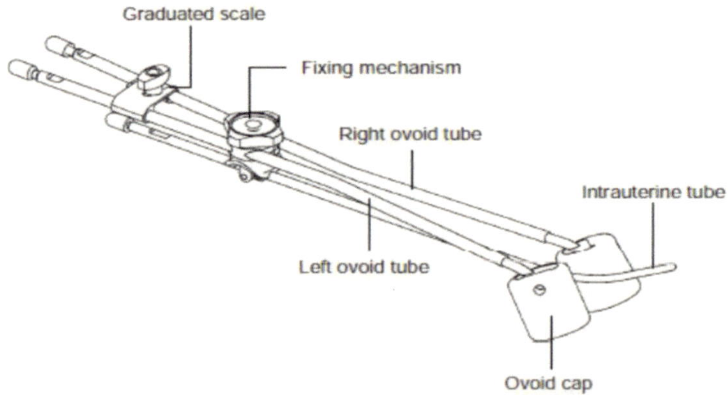

Figure 6.
Fletcher Williamson applicator.

was defined as 5 mm behind the posterior vaginal wall, which was localized with the help of a rectal retractor containing radiopaque material. In addition to these points, the dose to two other points, which are 1.5 cm superior and inferior to the ICRU bladder points should also be recorded. In a study by Srivastava et al. [45], it was observed that the dose at a point 1.5 cm above the ICRU bladder point was higher than the ICRU bladder point dose. This means that the ICRU bladder point is not the true representation of the maximum point dose to the bladder (**Figure 7**). A three-dimensional pear-shaped isodose distribution is obtained and displayed in the TPS. A dose of 7 Gy per fraction for three fractions is prescribed in brachytherapy treatment. Optimization is done by changing dwell positions in plans where bladder or rectum doses are observed to be high. These plans are then exported to the treatment console for treatment on a brachytherapy machine.

Treatment planning on 2D images, however, has limitations. The target volume could not be delineated, so the clinical target volume (CTV) covered by the reference isodose could not be identified. Moreover, maximum doses to the organs at risk, such

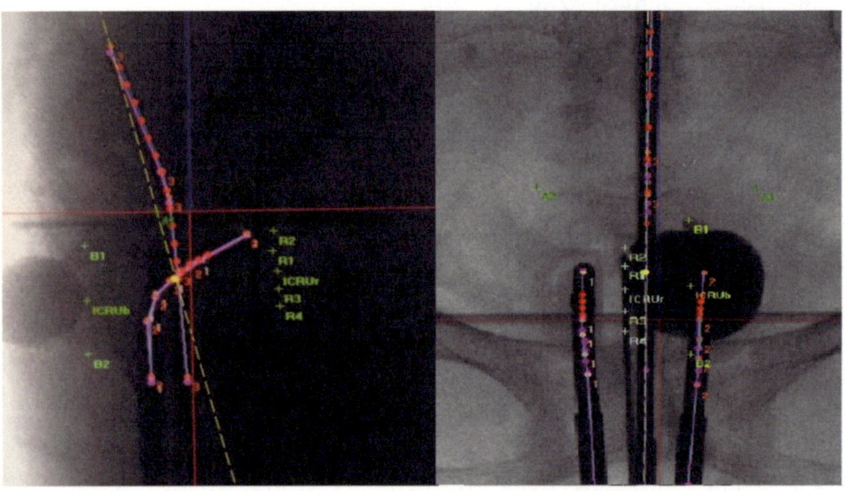

Figure 7.
Lateral and AP radiograph showing ICRU bladder and ICRU rectum point.

as bladder and rectum, could not be evaluated as 2D image-based treatment planning gave information about only the point doses to these OARs, which was insufficient to predict the toxicities. This gave path to the need to express dose distribution in three dimensions (3D), giving rise to the emergence of 3D image-based brachytherapy.

4.3.2 Three-dimensional image-based brachytherapy

In earlier decades, two-dimensional imaging (orthogonal radiographs) was widely used for treatment planning in brachytherapy. This treatment planning method provided limited information about the tumor dimensions and dose to the target and OARs. Since this method relied on point-based dose prescription, it resulted in under dosage in case of bulky tumors and overdosage in small tumors. With the advent of 3D imaging modalities like CT, MRI and USG, knowing the true extent of a tumor has become easy. 3D imaging helps in tumor volume assessment and delineation of OARs.

Image-based brachytherapy gives a basis for understanding the relationship between absorbed dose and volume. 3D image-based planning helps in the evaluation of dose-volume parameters and their correlation with clinical results. It is useful for individualization of dose distribution as per patient's anatomy and tumor extent with the help of the information obtained from the dose-volume histogram (DVH). This helps improve the coverage of the target and reduce the dose to OARs.

In 2005, recommendations on terms and parameters used in 3D image-based brachytherapy were published by the GYN GEC-ESTRO Working Group, which emphasized the use of sectional imaging for tumor volume assessment. After a year, the Working Group developed another guideline that focused on 3D dose-volume parameters in treatment planning. Instead of point, the volume-based prescription was used, and dose to target and OARs were evaluated in terms of these dose-volume parameters [46, 47].

Image-based brachytherapy has several benefits, which include knowing the tumor extent clearly, target-based prescription instead of a point-based prescription, evaluation of dose received by tumor and OARs, and optimizing the dose when necessary verifying the position of applicators and facility to use interstitial brachytherapy in combination with intracavitary brachytherapy.

Two CTVs are recommended for delineation in brachytherapy of the cervix. The first target is defined based on GTV at the time of diagnosis, called as intermediate risk CTV, to which a dose of 60 Gy is prescribed. The second target is defined based on GTV at the time of brachytherapy, known as High-Risk CTV. A dose of 80–90 Gy is prescribed to the second target. Dose-volume parameters for target volumes and OARs can be obtained from cumulative dose volume histogram (DVH) analysis in the 3D image-based treatment plan. The parameters for the target are the minimum dose delivered to 100% volume (D100) and 90% of the volume of interest (D90), respectively, and the volume enclosed by 100% of the prescribed dose. For OARs, parameters D2cc, D1cc and D0.1cc representing minimum dose to maximum irradiated tissue volumes of 2 cc, 1 cc and 0.1 cc are evaluated from DVH.

In three-dimensional ICRT planning, 3D images like CT and MRI are used. Patients undergo CT or MRI after the ICRT application. These images are then transferred to TPS for contouring and planning. CTV and OARs like bladder, rectum and bowel are delineated. After the delineation, applicator reconstruction and source loading are done. A dose of 7 Gy per fraction for three fractions is prescribed. The dose to target and OARs are calculated using the dose calculation algorithm in the TPS. A three-dimensional pear-shaped isodose distribution is obtained and displayed

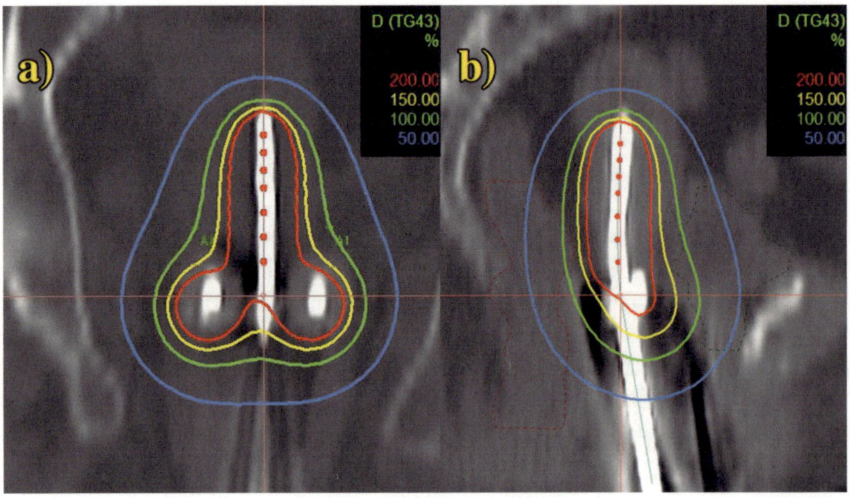

Figure 8.
Isodose distribution of an ICBT patient in (a) coronal view (b) sagittal view.

in the TPS (**Figure 8**). DVH parameters of the CTV, including D90, V100 and D100 and of the OARs, including D2cc, D1cc and D0.1cc, are evaluated from DVH. The plans are optimized for good target coverage and reduced OAR doses. These plans are then exported to the treatment console for treatment on a brachytherapy machine.

5. Toxicities of radiotherapy

Estimates of the risk of late complications of radical radiotherapy vary according to the grading system, duration of follow-up, method of calculation, treatment method, and prevalence of risk factors in the study population. However, most reports quote an overall risk of significant complications (requiring transfusion, hospitalization, or surgical intervention) of 5 to 15%. Complication rates may be higher in patients with very locally advanced disease partly because of tissue destruction caused by an infiltrative tumor.

Acute: During pelvic radiotherapy, most patients have mild fatigue and mild-to-moderate diarrhea that usually is controllable with antidiarrheal medications; some patients have mild bladder irritation, which may be symptomatic of a urinary tract infection. When extended fields are treated, patients may have nausea, gastric irritation, and depression of peripheral blood cell counts. Haematologic and gastrointestinal complications are significantly increased in patients receiving concurrent chemotherapy. Unless the ovaries have been transposed, all premenopausal patients who receive pelvic radiotherapy experience ovarian failure by the completion of treatment.

Perioperative complications of intracavitary brachytherapy include uterine perforation, fever and the usual risks of anesthesia.

Late: During the first 3 years after treatment, rectal complications (Radiation proctitis) are most common and include bleeding, stricture, ulceration and fistula. In the study by Eifel et al. [7], the risk of major rectosigmoid complications was 2.3% at 5 years. Major gastrointestinal complications were rare 3 years or more after treatment, but a constant low risk of urinary tract complications persisted for many years. The actuarial risk of developing a fistula of any type was 1.7% at 5 years. Small bowel obstruction is an infrequent complication of standard radiotherapy for patients without special risk factors.

Numerous psychological and physical factors can influence sexual function after pelvic radiation therapy. Most patients who received definitive radiation therapy for cervical cancer have some telangiectasia of the apical vagina. More significant vaginal shortening can occur, particularly in elderly, postmenopausal women and those with extensive tumors treated with a high radiation dose. Hypoestrogenism can enhance vaginal atrophy and dryness, contributing to dyspareunia. Intravaginal or systemic estrogen may reduce these symptoms. Vaginal dilatation and vaginal dilation may help prevent vaginal stenosis or improve quality of life.

6. Conclusion

Cervical carcinoma is the fourth most common malignancy in women worldwide, and it is most prevalent in Asia, Africa, and Central and South America. Radiotherapy plays a significant role in managing cervical cancer, with the standard mode of definitive treatment in locally advanced cervical carcinoma patients.

EBRT is part of the routine treatment of cervical carcinoma, targeting the draining lymph nodal groups and, in some cases, the para-aortic or inguinal group of lymph nodes. Intensity-Modulated Radiation Therapy (IMRT) is now recommended for EBRT due to its potential to reduce treatment-related toxicities and improve survival. Image-guided Radiotherapy (IGRT) is recommended along with IMRT/VMAT to limit PTV margins and ensure safe dose delivery. IMRT/VMAT can also safely deliver boost doses to pathological pelvic or para-aortic lymph nodes safely.

External beam radiotherapy along with brachytherapy is the standard treatment for cervical cancer with FIGO staging IIB-IIIB. The most common brachytherapy technique used in the treatment of cervical cancer is intracavitary brachytherapy, but in cases where intracavitary techniques are not feasible, interstitial brachytherapy is used. Image-based brachytherapy planning has emerged as a solution to the limitations of 2D image-based treatment planning. Image-based planning helps evaluate dose-volume parameters and their correlation with clinical results, improving tumor coverage and reducing the dose to organs at risk. Toxicities of radiotherapy vary according to the grading system, duration of follow-up, method of calculation, treatment method and prevalence of risk factors in the study population.

Author details

Shraddha Srivastava[1*], Nara Singh Moirangthem[2], Arunima Ghosh[1], Indrajeet Gupta[1] and Madan Lal Brahma Bhatt[1]

1 Department of Radiotherapy, King George's Medical University, Lucknow, India

2 Department of Radiation Oncology, Dr. B. Borooah Cancer Institute, Guwahati, India

*Address all correspondence to: shraddha686@gmail.com

References

[1] Sung H, Ferlay J, Siegel RL, Laversanne M, Soerjomataram I, Jemal A, et al. Global cancer statistics 2020: GLOBOCAN estimates of incidence and mortality worldwide for 36 cancers in 185 countries. CA: A Cancer Journal for Clinicians. 2021;**71**(3):209-249

[2] Mathur P, Sathishkumar K, Chaturvedi M, Das P, Sudarshan KL, Santhappan S, et al. Cancer statistics, 2020: Report from National Cancer Registry Programme, India. JCO Global Oncology. 2020;**6**:1063-1075

[3] Hochman A, Ratzkowski E, Schreiber H. Incidence of carcinoma of the cervix in Jewish women in Israel. British Journal of Cancer. 1955;**9**(3):358-364

[4] Bosch FX, Lorincz A, Munoz N, et al. The causal relation between human papillomavirus and cervical cancer. Journal of Clinical Pathology. 2002;**55**:244-265

[5] Tanderup K, Eifel PJ, Yashar CM, Pötter R, Grigsby PW. Curative radiation therapy for locally advanced cervical cancer: Brachytherapy is NOT optional. International Journal of Radiation Oncology, Biology, Physics. 2014;**88**(3):537-539

[6] Viswanathan AN, Erickson B, Gaffney DK, Beriwal S, Bhatia SK, Lee BO. Comparison and consensus guidelines for delineation of clinical target volume for CT and MR-based brachytherapy in locally advanced cervical cancer. International Journal of Radiation Oncology, Biology, Physics. 2014;**90**(2):320-328

[7] Eifel PJ, Morris M, Wharton JT, et al. The influence of tumor size and morphology on the outcome of patients with FIGO stage IB squamous cell carcinoma of the uterine cervix. International Journal of Radiation Oncology, Biology, Physics. 1994;**29**(1):9-16

[8] Keys HM, Bundy BN, Stehman FB, Muderspach LI, Chafe WE, Suggs CL, et al. Cisplatin, radiation, and adjuvant hysterectomy compared with radiation and adjuvant hysterectomy for bulky stage IB cervical carcinoma. New England Journal of Medicine. 1999;**340**(15):1154-1161

[9] Peters WA, Liu PY, Barrett RJ, et al. Concurrent chemotherapy and pelvic radiation therapy compared with pelvic radiation therapy alone as adjuvant therapy after radical surgery in high-risk early-stage cancer of the cervix. Journal of Clinical Oncology. 2000;**18**:1606-1613

[10] Whitney CW, Sause W, Bundy BN, et al. Randomized comparison of fluorouracil plus cisplatin versus hydroxyurea as an adjunct to radiation therapy in stage IIB-IVA carcinoma of the cervix with negative Para-aortic lymph nodes: A Gynecologic oncology group and southwest oncology group study. Journal of Clinical Oncology. 1999;**17**:1339-1338

[11] Rose PG, Bundy BN, Watkins EB, et al. Concurrent cisplatin-based radiotherapy and chemotherapy for locally advanced cervical cancer. The New England Journal of Medicine. 1999;**340**:1144-1143

[12] Chino J, Annunziata CM, Beriwal S, Bradfield L, Erickson BA, Fields EC, et al. The ASTRO clinical practice guidelines in cervical cancer: Optimizing radiation therapy for improved outcomes. Gynecologic Oncology. 2020;**159**:607-610

[13] Cibula D, Raspollini MR, Planchamp F, Centeno C, Chargari C,

Felix A, et al. ESGO/ESTRO/ESP guidelines for the management of patients with cervical cancer - Update 2023. International Journal of Gynecological Cancer. 2023;**33**:649-666

[14] Toita T, Ohno T, Kaneyasu Y, Kato T, Uno T, Hatano K, et al. A consensus-based guideline defining clinical target volume for primary disease in external beam radiotherapy for intact uterine cervical cancer. Japanese Journal of Clinical Oncology. 2011;**41**:1119-1126

[15] Bansal A, Patel F, Rai B, Gulia A, Dhanireddy B, Sharma S. Literature review with PGI guidelines for delineation of clinical target volume for intact carcinoma cervix. Journal of Cancer Research and Therapeutics. 2013;**9**:574-582

[16] Small W, Bosch WR, Harkenrider MM, Strauss JB, Abu-Rustum N, Albuquerque KV, et al. NRG oncology/RTOG consensus guidelines for delineation of clinical target volume for intensity modulated pelvic radiation therapy in postoperative treatment of endometrial and cervical cancer: An update. International Journal of Radiation Oncology, Biology, Physics. 2021;**109**:413-424

[17] Sedlis A, Bundy BN, Rotman MZ, Lentz SS, Muderspach LI, Zaino RJ. A randomized trial of pelvic radiation therapy versus No further therapy in selected patients with stage IB carcinoma of the cervix after radical hysterectomy and pelvic lymphadenectomy: A Gynecologic oncology group study. Gynecologic Oncology. 1999;**73**:177-183

[18] International Atomic Energy Agency. Management of Cervical Cancer: Strategies for Limited-Resource Centres-A Guide for Radiation Oncologists. IAEA Human Health Reports No. 6. Vienna: IAEA; 2013

[19] Nishimura Y, Komaki R. Intensity-modulated Radiation Therapy: Clinical Evidence and Techniques. 1st ed. Tokyo: Springer; 2015

[20] Lin AJ, Kidd E, Dehdashti F, Siegel BA, Mutic S, Thaker PH, et al. Intensity modulated radiation therapy and image-guided adapted brachytherapy for cervix cancer HHS public access. International Journal of Radiation Oncology, Biology, Physics. 2019;**103**:1088-1097

[21] Chang Y, Yang ZY, Li GL, Li Q, Yang Q, Fan JQ, et al. Correlations between radiation dose in bone marrow and Hematological toxicity in patients with cervical cancer: A comparison of 3DCRT, IMRT, and RapidARC. International Journal of Gynecological Cancer. 2016;**26**:770-776

[22] Cho B. Intensity-modulated radiation therapy: A review with a physics perspective. Radiation Oncology Journal. 2018;**36**:1-10

[23] Chopra S, Gupta S, Kannan S, Dora T, Engineer R, Mangaj A, et al. Late toxicity after adjuvant conventional radiation versus image-guided intensity-modulated radiotherapy for cervical cancer (PARCER): A randomized controlled trial. Journal of Clinical Oncology. 2021;**39**:3682-3692

[24] Lin Y, Chen K, Lu Z, Zhao L, Tao Y, Ouyang Y, et al. Intensity-modulated radiation therapy for definitive treatment of cervical cancer: A meta-analysis. Radiation Oncology. 2018;**13**:177

[25] Viswanathan AN, Thomadsen B. American brachytherapy society consensus guidelines for locally advanced carcinoma of the cervix. Part I: General principles. Brachytherapy. 2012;**11**:33-46

[26] Vale C, Tierney JF, Stewart LA, Brady M, Dinshaw K, Jakobsen A, et al. Reducing uncertainties about the effects

of Chemoradiotherapy for cervical cancer: A systematic review and meta-analysis of individual patient data from 18 randomized trials. Journal of Clinical Oncology. 2008;**26**:5802

[27] Gerbaulet A, Ash D, Meertens H. General aspects. In: Gerbaulet A, Pötter R, Mazeron JJ, Meertens H, Limbergen EV, editors. The GEC ESTRO Handbook of Brachytherapy. Brussels: ACCO, ESTRO; 2002. pp. 1-7

[28] Tod M, Meredith WJ. Treatment of cancer of the cervix uteri, a revised Manchester method. The British Journal of Radiology. 1953;**26**(305):252-257

[29] Chassagne D, Horiot JC. Proposals for common definitions of reference points in gynaecological brachytherapy. Journal of Radiology and Nuclear Medicine. 1977;**58**(5):371-373

[30] Haas JS, Dean RD, Mansfield CM. Evaluation of a new fletcher applicator using Cesium-137. International Journal of Radiation Oncology* Biology* Physics. 1980;**6**(11):1589-1595

[31] Podgorsak EB. Radiation Oncology Physics: A Handbook for Teachers and Students. Vienna: IAEA; 2015

[32] Singh MN, Kinhikar RA, Agarwal JP, Laskar SG. Principles and practice of radiation oncology. In: Kataki AC, Barmon D, editors. Fundamentals in Gynaecologic Malignancy. Singapore: Springer; 2022

[33] Blake P. Clinical introduction to brachytherapy. In: Mayles P, Nahum A, Rosenwald JC, editors. Handbook of Radiotherapy and Physics: Theory and Practice. London: Taylor and Francis group: CRC Press; 2007. pp. 1094-1096

[34] Nag S. High dose rate brachytherapy: Its clinical applications and treatment guidelines. Technology in Cancer Research & Treatment. 2004;**3**(3):269-287

[35] Atahan IL, Onal C, Ozyar E, Yiliz F, Selek U, Kose F. Long-term outcome and prognostic factors in patients with cervical carcinoma: A retrospective study. International Journal of Gynecological Cancer. 2007;**17**(4):833-842

[36] Viani GA, Manta GB, Stefano EJ, de Fendi LI. Brachytherapy for cervix cancer: Low dose rate or high-dose rate brachytherapy–A meta-analysis of clinical trials. Journal of Experimental & Clinical Cancer Research. 2009;**28**(1):47

[37] Montana GS, Hanlon AL, Brickner TJ, Owen JB, Hanks GE, Ling CC, et al. Carcinoma of the cervix: Patterns of care studies: Review of 1978, 1983, and 1988-1989 surveys. International Journal of Radiation Oncology*Biology*Physics. 1995;**32**(5):1481-1486

[38] Lanciano RM, Martz K, Coia LR, Hanks GE. Tumor and treatment factors improving outcome in stage III-B cervix cancer. International Journal of Radiation Oncology, Biology, Physics. 1991;**20**(1):95-100

[39] Srivastava S, Singh N, Varghese M. Determination of variation in dosimetric parameters of treatment planning with Co-60 and Ir-192 sources in high dose rate brachytherapy of cervical carcinoma. Radiation Physics and Chemistry. 2022;**196**:110148

[40] Srivastava S, Singh N, Kashyap VK. Optimization methods in interstitial brachytherapy: A comparative study of inverse planning simulated annealing with graphical optimization and geometrical optimization in cervical cancer. Journal of Biomedical Physics and Engineering. 2022;**12**(4):339-348

[41] Leung S. Perineal template techniques for interstitial implantation of gynaecological cancers using the Paris system of dosimetry. International Journal of Radiation Oncology, Biology, Physics. 1990;**19**(3):769-774

[42] Erickson B, Albano K, Gillin M. CT-guided interstitial implantation of gynaecologic malignancies. International Journal of Radiation Oncology, Biology, Physics. 1996;**36**(3):699-709

[43] Martinez A, Cox RS, Edmunson GK. A multiple site perineal applicator (MUPIT) for treatment of prostatic, anorectal and gynecological malignancies. International Journal of Radiation Oncology, Biology, Physics. 1984;**10**(2):297-305

[44] International Commission on Radiological Units. Dose and Volume Specification for Reporting Intracavitary Therapy in Gynecology. Report No 38. Washington DC: ICRU Publications; 1985

[45] Srivastava S, Painuly NK, Mishra SP, Srivastava K, Singh N, Singh S, et al. Evaluation of volumetric doses of organs at risk in carcinoma cervix patients with HDR intracavitary brachytherapy and comparison of CT-based and conventional plans. Journal of Biomedical Physics and Engineering. 2019;**9**(6):603-612

[46] Haie-Meder C, Pötter R, Van Limbergen E, Briot E, De Brabandere M, Dimopoulos J, et al. Recommendations from gynaecological (GYN) GEC-ESTRO working group* (I): Concepts and terms in 3D image-based 3D treatment planning in cervix cancer brachytherapy with emphasis on MRI assessment of GTV and CTV. Radiotherapy and Oncology. 2005;**74**(3):235-245

[47] Pötter R, Haie-Meder C, Van Limbergen E, Barillot I, De Brabandere M, Dimopoulos J, et al. Recommendations from gynaecological (GYN) GEC ESTRO working group (II): Concepts and terms in 3D image-based treatment planning in cervix cancer brachytherapy—3D dose-volume parameters and aspects of 3D image-based anatomy, radiation physics, radiobiology. Radiotherapy and Oncology. 2006;**78**(1):67-77

Chapter 3

The Costs of Cervical Cancer Treatment with a Social Focus

Johanna Melissa Aguayo Joza, Carlos Javier Más López, Guido Enrique Terán Mogro, Luis Santiago Quiroz Fernández, Shirley Elizabeth Pizarro Anchundia, Amy Melissa Loor Aguayo and Joan Manuel Loor Aguayo

Abstract

The study of the value creation system in the strategic management of costs associated with diseases shows the need to focus the analysis on the activities that make it up, since they detail all the interrelated actions to achieve efficiency in their treatment, particularly in cervical cancer. The design of its value chain is important in the economic context in which it is created and the agents involved in its achievement, since the user, the provider and the financer of health care have different health, economic and political interests. Quantifying its economic impact on society is relevant for its economic evaluation, reducing uncertainty and optimizing the design of public policies. There are theoretical and methodological weaknesses in the methods for estimating their indirect costs, market imperfections and the postulates of economic theory as their main foundations. The objective of the article is to design the value chain of the disease and the calculation of its costs, which will be specified by highlighting which activities will be considered as contributing value to its treatments and which others will be considered as supporting activities for the beneficiary of its treatments, who will be the patient.

Keywords: cervical cancer, value chain, direct costs of disease, indirect disease costs, unit cost of illness

1. Introduction

The International Union Against Cancer diagnoses twelve million people worldwide each year and 7.6 million die from cervical cancer. In Latin America, this disease is the second leading cause of death in women, especially affecting the lower socioeconomic levels [1].

Cervical cancer, or cancer of the cervix, is a disease in which cancerous (malignant) cells are found in the tissues of the cervix. It develops slowly, beginning with a precancerous lesion called dysplasia. The most frequent cause of cervical cancer is the human papillomavirus (HPV), which is transmitted through sexual intercourse [2]. In Ecuador for some years, it has been one of the leading causes of death among women.

This disease, like many others, requires a large expenditure of resources on the part of both state and private health authorities. Managing them within the institutions that provide health services, while respecting their characteristics, becomes an important challenge for this type of organization.

1.1 The direct cost of disease treatment

The cost of treatment of diseases is a partial evaluation within health economic evaluations; these types of studies analyze the direct health and non-health costs generated by these, as well as the indirect costs associated with them [3–5].

However, after a review of several of these studies, it was determined that there was no standard methodology for the treatment of costs associated with the disease and essentially classifying them in terms of the object of costs—the disease—into direct and indirect [4, 5].

This problem is coupled with the fact that there are two points of view on how to cost illness: one approach taken from the treatment given by accountants, using concepts from management accounting, and another from the vision held by health economists who essentially differ in the treatment that indirect costs receive. However, the authors acknowledge after an extensive literature search that a large majority of these studies use the health economists' version of the cost of illness [5, 6].

In many studies, direct health costs are estimated by multiplying a vector of quantities of resources consumed by a vector of prices [7, 8]. For this purpose, both vectors are constructed by considering all the inputs used in the care process and the market prices associated with each one, respectively. Among the resources commonly considered, some authors [9, 10] highlight outpatient care, medical consultation, hospitalization costs, medication and laboratory tests, as well as resources consumed in emergency services, nursing homes and home care. However, other authors also consider those resources consumed in rehabilitation and specialized care [11–13].

Likewise, direct non-health costs include the expenses of patients, relatives, friends and non-profit institutions in terms of payments for transportation, food, hygienization, caregivers, medications and other inputs borne by these agents [14]. In order to value them correctly and obtain satisfactory results in their management, it becomes necessary to broaden the range of analysis, from the formation of their value chain to the information resulting from the calculation of their costs [15–17].

One of the main problems in cost-of-illness studies is the distribution of indirect costs to direct activities, since most studies on this subject are devoted to adding up independently both direct health and non-health costs and the indirect costs associated with these [4].

In addition to these elements, health care nowadays has become a market where various health care providers are present and compete to obtain a larger number of clients. This strategic competition ranges from having better trained human resources, medical procedures with the latest advances in medical sciences to efficient cost management that provides a target cost necessary to maintain an expected profit margin [4].

Hence, health care institutions must borrow three essential elements from the strategic management of business systems: achieving strategic positioning in health care markets, designing value chains for key factors such as disease and managing their costs efficiently associated with the activities that generate value in their treatments.

1.2 The disease treatment value chain

The design of the disease treatment value chain is a novel element in its management. It is recognized as the interrelated double value chain, which links both healthcare and non-healthcare activities in the conception and delivery of value that makes it possible to achieve efficiency in the use of human, technological and material resources, resulting in the improvement of the quality of life of patients or in their definitive cure [6, 18].

The health chain of the disease has as by all the supplies that companies focused or not on health services provide, i.e., medical, primary care and indirect supplies to the health service [6, 19].

Direct health activities are the medical procedures that directly influence the provision of services in the entity, such as outpatient consultations, hospitalization, diagnostic tests, among others. The support activities help the main activities to develop satisfactorily, including the actions carried out by the administrative development department, where the areas of planning, accounting, finance, investment management, human resources management, technological development, purchasing and supply, among others, are grouped together [6, 19].

The non-health value chain of cervical cancer treatment, as for many other diseases, includes all the costs, skills and knowledge that social agents such as family members, friends and non-profit institutions contribute to improving the quality of life of patients afflicted with this disease within a given social environment (14,18] [20–22]. This disease, it integrates social values, which are nothing more than human values that are part of the social culture such as ethics, morality, solidarity, humanity, survival, etc., with the costs borne by patients, families, friends and social organizations, state prevention policies, the medical culture of the population and ancestral knowledge and with the beneficiaries of the services, the patients.

This value chain is composed of core and support activities linked to the social agents that support the disease. Among the main activities are expenditures for transportation, food, sanitation, payments to caregivers and other activities carried out by families, friends and non-profit institutions involved in improving the quality of life of patients. Support activities include activities that describe the results of policies for the prevention of cervical cancer carried out by health authorities and other social organizations, the activities they develop, the medical culture and the patient-health institution relationship, as well as the ancestral knowledge of the population that has survived from generation to generation regarding the treatment of this ailment [6, 19].

The margin of advantage in the fight against cervical cancer treatments could be understood as the contribution of value generated by all the main activities within its value chain as well as the value that emerges in the relationships between them that should guarantee efficiency in the use of available resources by the social agents as well as the design of policies by the state in terms of decreasing the incidence of this disease on the agents involved [6, 19].

Now, having an adequate design of the value chain, for any process, contributes to developing a cost leadership strategy that allows the achievement of efficiency and savings of all types of resources [23, 24], but which cost system will be the most appropriate to achieve the organization's strategies?

Traditional systems have the disadvantage of not providing sufficient information for decision-making, they only use quantitative data, they emphasize production or service costs and they use limited criteria for the distribution of indirect costs, which makes it necessary to use other procedures that meet current information needs for management and decision making [6, 23–26].

To solve these problems, Activity Based Costing (ABC) and Activity Based Management (ABM) have emerged, although their design and application predate the development of the conceptualization of the value chain, the authors agree with the specialists consulted [6, 23–29] that the analysis of the value chain makes it easier for the organization to define a better structure by activities.

It is necessary to emphasize that the objective of this article is to design the value chain of the disease and the calculation of its costs, so it will be specified in highlighting which activities will be considered as value contributors to their treatments and which others will be considered as support for the beneficiary of their treatments, who will be the patient. In the same way, the procedure to cost their activities and some relevant elements in their illustration in SOLCA Manabí, Portoviejo, Ecuador, is presented.

2. Materials and methods

2.1 Research universe

A retrospective-descriptive cross-sectional study was conducted in 2016, measuring the prevalence of exposure of patients and their expenses associated with cervical cancer, family members, friends and their outcomes (treatment costs) in the period that the study was developed.

A total of 189 records were reviewed, which were all the patients attended in one year, having been necessary the design of an annotation sheet per patient. It should be noted that in the case of SOLCA Manabí, Núcleo de Portoviejo, the patient's logbook (clinical history) is in a database where the physician updates the information resulting from all the medical procedures undergone by the patient, an element that greatly facilitates the statistical work. In addition, a survey was carried out to determine the costs associated with the disease for 122 people, including 61 patients suffering from cervical cancer, 46 family members and 15 friends.

2.2 The cervical cancer value chain

The cervical cancer treatment value chain consists of two chains that complement each other (**Figure 1**): a health chain and a non-health chain. The two chains are linked together and show the activities that add value to the treatments for the disease.

2.2.1 Health care value chain for cervical cancer treatments

First, the design of the chain required a representation of each link in the process using the relevant techniques for this case, such as a bibliographic study and the expertise of the working group or other specialists when necessary to define the hierarchies of the processes, especially the disease protocol.

Following the sequence of the tasks described above, the input of the chain is composed of both state and private companies, mainly from the province of Manabí and its neighbor Guayas, mainly from its capital Guayaquil, which provides primary care medical supplies for the health service, companies such as Simed, Magnamedical, Sumelab, Ecuador Overseas, among others.

To define the main activities, outpatient consultations, hospitalization and clinical laboratory were established, including DNA testing for Human Papilloma Virus

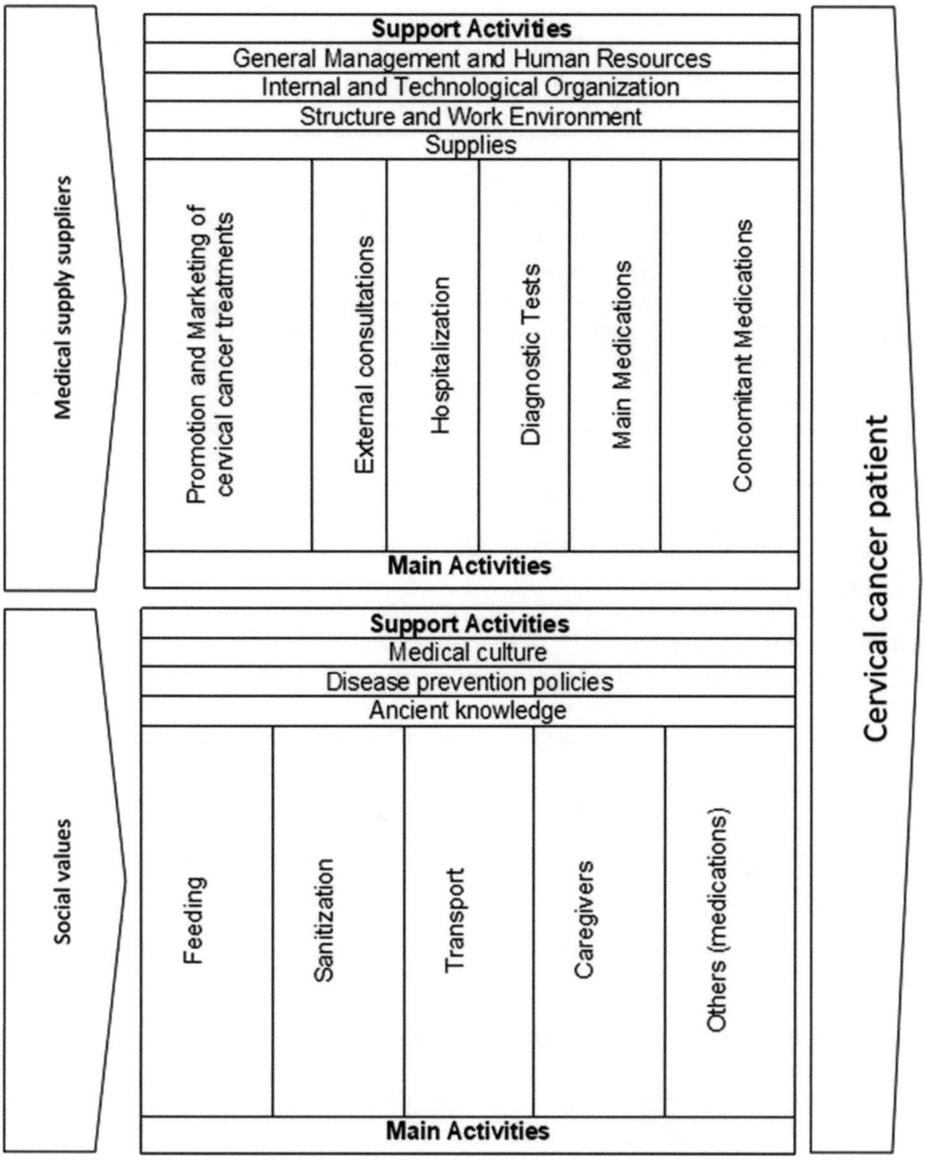

Figure 1.
Value chain of cervical cancer treatments in SOLCA, Manabí. Source: Adapted from Michel Potter from his book "Competitive Advantage" [30].

(HPV), vaginal autotomy, Papanicolaou screening (Pap smear), among others; and oncological medical procedures such as radiotherapy and chemotherapy.

Among the support activities are the actions carried out by the administrative development department, which includes the areas of planning, accounting, finance, investment management, human resources administration, technological development, purchasing and supply, among others.

The output of the health value chain is the interrelationships of the main activities (outpatient consultations, hospitalization, diagnostic tests and medical procedures for oncology patients) with their support activities (administrative, logistic, etc.)

that allow an advantage in the application of the treatment for the improvement of the quality of life of patients with cervical cancer. The beneficiaries of the healthcare value chain are the patients with this type of ailment.

2.2.2 Non-healthcare value chain of cervical cancer treatments

The inputs of the cervical cancer non-health value chain were defined by social values prevalent in society such as love of family, solidarity and humanity.

The main activities in the cervical cancer non-health value chain were essentially defined by food, sanitation, transportation, caregivers and drugs.

Support activities were identified with the medical culture acquired by patients, family and friends, as well as with the result of the prevention policies of the health authorities against cervical cancer; and, with the ancestral knowledge transmitted from generation to generation that favors the improvement of health.

2.3 Procedure

The procedure for calculating the health and non-health costs that determined the total cost of cervical cancer treatments was based on the financial statements of the selected entity and the expenses of its patients, family members and friends associated with their treatments.

The following tasks were carried out to determine the health costs of treatment:

1. Select the key direct and indirect areas of responsibility or sub-areas of health services.

2. Make the secondary distribution of indirect costs from the support areas to the direct areas in the provision of health services, selecting the appropriate basis for their allocation.

3. Calculate the rates of indirect expenses of the direct areas to the provision of services.

4. Calculate the unit costs of medical procedures.

    - The total number in each area of responsibility or key sub-area with its total allocated costs was taken.

    - The corresponding distribution coefficient or other appropriate method was determined and multiplied by the number of specific procedures to obtain their unit costs.

    - The unit costs were multiplied by the units of measure (cost drivers) for each activity per patient.

5. Calculate sanitary costs for each direct activity.

6. Determine the costs by health stages of cervical cancer.

7. Calculate the total health care costs of cervical cancer treatments.

8. Calculate the average unit health costs per patient.

The following steps were taken to determine non-health costs:

1. Develop and apply a questionnaire to obtain the information necessary to determine the costs of direct non-health activities:

    - Make a selection of the patients, family members and/or friends involved in the selected time period.

    - Collect the information needed to prepare the questionnaire.

    - Prepare and apply the questionnaire to calculate the costs of non-health activities.

2. Calculate non-health costs for each direct activity designed.

    - Calculate the non-health costs of each direct activity per respondent.

3. Calculate the coefficient of salaries of patients, relatives and friends involved in the research and indirect non-health expenses.

    - Obtain the salary of patients, relatives and friends.

    - Calculate the salary coefficients of patients, relatives and friends.

    - Calculate non-health indirect costs.

4. Define cost drivers to allocate non-health indirect costs.

    - Define the cost drivers for each of the direct non-health activities.

5. Distribute indirect costs to direct non-health activities.

6. Estimate the non-health costs of cervical cancer treatments.

7. Calculation of total and unit costs of cervical cancer treatments.

In addition, as a relevant element, the cost per stage of the treatment of the disease is shown, taking into account the approved protocols [31].

- Stage 0 (In situ): In situ cases with carcinomas that are cured only with the cone leep and periodic check-ups, do not require further treatment for cure.

- Stage 1: The disease is limited to the cervix only.

- Stage 2: It goes beyond the cervix, but does not affect the pelvic wall or the lower third of the vagina.

- Stage 3: There is an incidence in the pelvic wall and/or involvement of the lower third of the vagina and/or causes hydroureteronephrosis or renal failure.

- Stage 4: There is already metastasis or involvement of other organs such as bladder, rectum, lung, liver and brain.

It is important to note that the study was approved by SOLCA's Board of Directors, which determined its scope and the time horizon of the research. Its results were discussed and are presented below.

3. Results

As indicated above, the costs of cervical cancer treatments at SOLCA Manabí, Portoviejo, Ecuador, were calculated taking into account the expenses incurred by the entity in one year. The following tables (**Tables 1–3**) present the calculations derived from the application of the procedure. The total health care cost for the treatments was US$ 1,296,510.27, while the average unit cost per patient attended was US$ 6859.84.

The activities that generated the most expenses were hospitalization and outpatient consultation, respectively, while the activity that generated the least expenses was other oncological procedures.

Another element to highlight is that the stages of treatment that generated the most expenses were stages 3 and 4, which shows that these are the stages where most resources are allocated to treatment.

Tables 4–8 presents the calculations derived from the application of the procedure for non-health costs. The total non-health cost for the treatments was US$1,586,736.60, while the average non-health unit cost per patient attended was US$ 8395.43.

Total sanitary costs	
Direct activities	**Costs**
Outpatient	56.369,92
Hospitalization	1'170.742,70
Clinical laboratory	54.413,24
Other oncologic procedures	14.984,41
Total health care costs	1'296.510,27

Table 1.
Total health cost per activity of cervical cancer treatments.

Total unit sanitary costs	
Direct activities	**Costs**
Outpatient	298,25
Hospitalization	6.164,41
Clinical laboratory	287,90
Other oncologic procedures	78,28
Total sanitary average unit costs	6.859,84

Table 2.
Average unit health cost per activity of cervical cancer treatments.

Direct activities	Stage 0	Stage 1	Stage 2	Stage 3	Stage 4	Costs
Outpatient	14.360,30	2.188,24	2.598,53	15.299,17	25.929,48	56.369,92
Hospitalization	31.429,65	4.789,28	21.671,97	415.773,00	697.078,80	1'170.742,70
Clinical laboratory	20.210,87	4.637,19	10.405,93	12.978,53	6.180,72	54.413,24
Other oncologic procedures	3.817,30	581,68	690,75	4.066,92	5.827,76	14.984,41
Total costs per treatment stage	69.818,12	12.196,39	35.367,18	448.117,82	731.010,76	1'296.510,27

Table 3.
Cost by stages of health activities in the treatment of cervical cancer.

Main activities	Costs
Feeding	833.562,67
Transportation	114.074,67
Hygienization	116.162,47
Caregivers	48.605,83
Medications	202.270,83
Laboratories	247.336,17
Total	1'562.012,63

Table 4.
Direct non-health activities costs.

Activities	Activity-based cost drivers	Cost drivers
Feeding	Times of food consumption	1.157
Transportation	Times of transportation utilization	541
Hygienization	Number of toilets	10.411
Caregivers	Number of care	554
Medications	Number of doses	305
Laboratories	Number of tests	1.032

Table 5.
Non-sanitary cost drivers.

Once the health and non-health costs have been calculated, the tables (**Tables 9** and **10**) show the average total and unit costs for cervical cancer treatments. The total cost of treatments was US$2'883.246,87, while the average unit cost per patient treated was US$15.255,27.

Direct non-sanitary activities costs					
Main activities	**Costs**	**%**	**Indirect expenses**	**Cost drivers**	**Fees**
Feeding	833.562,67	0,533,646,559	13.193,86	1.157	11,4,035,104
Transportation	114.074,67	0,073030566	1.805,61	541	33,375,3331
Hygienization	116.162,47	0,074367175	1.838,65	10.411	0,17,660,665
Caregivers	48.605,83	0,031117439	769,35	554	13,887,1234
Medications	202.270,83	0,129,493,724	3.201,60	305	10,4,970,458
Laboratories	247.336,17	0,158,344,537	3.914,91	1.032	37,935,1315
Total	1'562.012,63	1,00	24.723,97		

Table 6.
Distribution of indirect non-health care expenses.

Main activities	Costs	Indirect expenses	Total direct non-health activities
Feeding	833.562,67	13.193,86	846.756,53
Transportation	114.074,67	1.805,61	115.880,27
Hygienization	116.162,47	1.838,65	118.001,12
Caregivers	48.605,83	769,35	49.375,18
Medications	202.270,83	3.201,60	205.472,43
Laboratories	247.336,17	3.914,91	251.251,07
Total	1'562.012,63	24.723,97	1'586.736,60

Table 7.
Total non-sanitary costs.

Main activities	Total direct non-health activities	Number of patients	Unit Cost
Feeding	846.756,53	189	4.480,19
Transportation	115.880,27	189	613,12
Hygienization	118.001,12	189	624,34
Caregivers	49.375,18	189	261,24
Medications	205.472,43	189	1.087,16
Laboratories	251.251,07	189	1.329,37
Total	1'586.736,60	189	8.395,43

Table 8.
Average non-sanitary unit costs per patient.

Total sanitary costs	Total non-sanitary costs	Total disease costs
1'296.510,27	1'586.736,60	2'883.246,87

Table 9.
Total costs of cervical cancer treatments.

Total disease costs	Total patients	Unit costs of disease
2'883.246,87	189	15.255,27

Table 10.
Average unit costs for cervical cancer treatment.

4. Discussion

The research determines the total and unit costs of cervical cancer treatment at SOLCA Manabí, Portoviejo, Ecuador. An essential element in the management of the costs associated with the treatment of the disease was the use of the value chain in its design, which made it possible to associate it with the activities that, according to its protocol, allow it to cope with the disease.

Although there are many studies that calculate the direct costs of the treatment of diseases in health institutions, those that use the tools of strategic cost management are limited. This is a novel approach within these types of studies since it is based on the idea that health services are provided in a healthcare market where there are several agents such as private, state or non-profit entities that compete for them.

Health services have a fundamental characteristic, which is that their ethical content of trying to save or maintain the quality of life of patients, regardless of the resources allocated to their treatment, should be the guiding principle. However, this ethical conflict is threatened in many cases by whether or not to provide patients with the necessary resources if they do not have health insurance to cover them.

This article is not intended to stir up controversy about health systems in many countries, but to show the tools of cost management to enable the efficiency of many providers of these services. Health is no stranger to the realities of the treatment of expenditures in many sectors of the economy and the calculation of the costs of their products or services. Traditional cost systems tend to overestimate or underestimate the costs of their products or services due to the defective treatment of the indirect costs associated with them. By managing them by activities, it is possible to correct them according to their cost generators, which make them more competitive, no matter the market where they are developed.

In the particular case of health services in the treatment of cervical cancer in SOLCA Manabí, Portoviejo, Ecuador, they have a particular treatment since it is a non-profit service provider. This does not mean that it does not need to make profits to invest in maintaining and increasing the quality of the services it provides. To this end, it charges the various insurances established in the Ecuadorian financial system the corresponding amounts according to the Tariff of benefits for the national health system approved by the Ministry of Public Health of Ecuador [32], so SOLCA, since it does not set the prices of the services, control of its costs will be objective in order to obtain the profit it requires, as shown in **Figure 2**.

It is important to clarify that, although the purpose of the research is not to design a tool to achieve a target cost, it can serve as a basis to achieve it, adapting to the realities of the environment of SOLCA Manabí, Núcleo de Portoviejo in setting the necessary utility for the quality of its services. Hence, the authors agree with Capasso [33] he states that the target cost "is not a costing methodology, it is a management tool that allows ordering, adapting and assembling the activities of the organization and its consequent costs to achieve a level of profitability in accordance with the objectives set by the management".

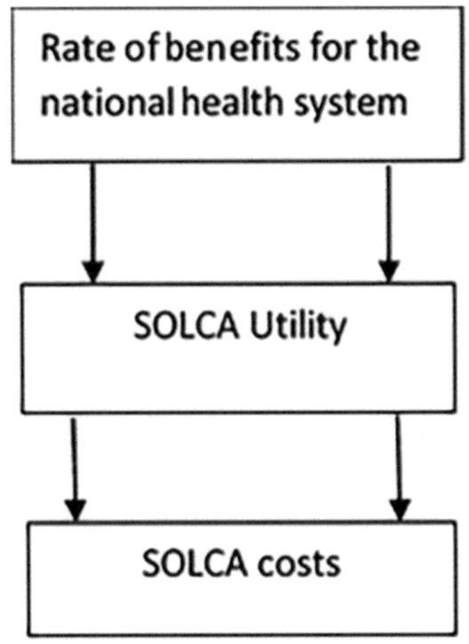

Figure 2.
Target costs in SOLCA.

In the same way, this procedure would serve as a basis for the control of the resources involved in cervical cancer treatments, since it would make it possible to detect deviations both in the costs of materials, personnel salaries and others directly or indirectly involved between their plan—the result that paid for the research—and the actual record in subsequent periods. The causes of these deviations should be detected and corrected to help achieve the organization's goals [19].

On the other hand, the calculation of non-health costs links health service providers with society, since its purpose is to assess the impact caused by the disease on patients, their families and other social agents. This will make it possible to articulate state policies that minimize the impact of the disease on the patients directly involved, not only for the health service providers but also for society as a whole [19].

To achieve an analysis of the results of non-health costs, the authors refer to the National Survey of Urban and Rural Household Income and Expenditures of Ecuador (ENIGHUR) where household expenditures are described for various items such as food and transportation, among others [34]. However, the last survey conducted was in 2011–2012 [35], well before the study presented here, so it was not possible to contrast the results of the research. The aim was to analyze the incidence of household expenses with those highlighted in the care of patients with cervical cancer.

But yes, with the data available in 2011–2012, it can be confirmed that since that date, food expenses have been the most relevant in Ecuadorian households with 24.40%, showing an increase in relation to previous studies [34], which reaffirms the authors' proposal. Hence, the results of non-health costs provide SOLCA Manabí, Núcleo de Portoviejo and the State, through its institutions, with a basis for assessing the impact of the disease on a relevant social sector such as women as essential members of Ecuadorian households.

5. Conclusions

Cervical cancer is a disease with a severe impact on the quality of life of the patients who suffer from it in many cases. The disease manifests itself with the appearance of cancerous (malignant) cells in the tissues of the cervix. It develops slowly, beginning with a precancerous lesion called dysplasia. The most common cause of cervical cancer is the human papillomavirus (HPV), which is transmitted through sexual intercourse. Cervical cancer can also impose a financial burden on healthcare systems. Although there are many studies that estimate the costs of treating disease in healthcare institutions, few use strategic cost management to determine these costs. This is a novel approach within these types of studies since it is based on the idea that the provision of health services is provided in a healthcare market where there are various agents such as private, state or non-profit entities that compete for it. In the same way, the inclusion of the non-health component in the costing methodology values the importance of the expenses of patients, their families and friends in achieving the quality of life of the patient with this ailment. It also provides relevant information for health authorities to propose state policies that minimize the impact of the disease on society through public policies. This study is an example of applying these tools in SOLCA Manabí, Portoviejo, Ecuador, which is trying to make the calculation of costs associated with cervical cancer treatments more efficient.

Acknowledgements

The authors thank the authorities of SOLCA for their support and the students of the Universidad Técnica de Manabí for their collaboration in the collection of data on the patients affected by this disease.

Authors' contributions

Johanna Melissa Aguayo Joza: Participated in the study and analysis of the conceptual elements related to the Introduction and Methodology. Contributed to the evaluation and discussion of the research results. Collaborated in the conclusions and bibliographical references.

Carlos Javier Más López: Participated in the study and analysis of the conceptual elements related to the Introduction and Methodology. Contributed to the evaluation and discussion of the research results. Collaborated in the conclusions and bibliographical references.

Guido Enrique Terán Mogro: Participated in the study and analysis of the conceptual elements related to the Introduction and Methodology. Contributed to the evaluation and discussion of the research results. Collaborated in the conclusions and bibliographical references.

Luis Santiago Quiroz Fernández: Participated in the study and analysis of the conceptual elements related to the Introduction and Methodology. Contributed to the evaluation and discussion of the research results. Collaborated in the conclusions and bibliographical references.

Shirley Elizabeth Pizarro Anchundia: Participated in the study and analysis of the conceptual elements related to the Introduction and Methodology. Contributed to the evaluation and discussion of the research results. Collaborated in the conclusions and bibliographical references.

Amy Melissa Loor Aguayo: Participated in the drafting and translation of the paper.

Joan Manuel Loor Aguayo: Participated in the study and analysis of the conceptual elements related to the Introduction and Methodology. Contributed to the evaluation and discussion of the research results. Collaborated in the conclusions and bibliographical references.

Conflict of interest

The authors declare that there are no conflicts of interest.

Author details

Johanna Melissa Aguayo Joza[1*], Carlos Javier Más López[2], Guido Enrique Terán Mogro[3], Luis Santiago Quiroz Fernández[4], Shirley Elizabeth Pizarro Anchundia[1], Amy Melissa Loor Aguayo[4] and Joan Manuel Loor Aguayo[4]

1 School of Administrative and Economic Sciences of the Universidad Técnica de Manabí, Portoviejo, Manabí, Ecuador

2 Faculty of Accounting and Finance, Department of Costs and Information Systems, University of Havana, Cuba

3 SOLCA Manabí, Núcleo de Portoviejo, Portoviejo, Manabí, Ecuador

4 Universidad Técnica de Manabí, Portoviejo, Manabí, Ecuador

*Address all correspondence to: johanna.aguayo@utm.edu.ec

References

[1] Roberts L. Unión Internacional Contra el Cáncer. Reino Unido. [Online]. 2020. Available from: https://www.telegraph.co.uk/global-health/science-and-disease/cervical-cancer-vaccine-boost-increases-supply-84-million-girls/

[2] Bansil P, Wittet S, Lim J, et al. Acceptability of self-collection sampling for HPV-DNA testing in low-resource settings: A mixed methods approach. BMC Public Health. 2014;**14**(596):2-9

[3] García Cáceres RG, Torres Valdivieso S, Ayala Escobar ÉS, Díaz Gómez HB, Vallejo Díaz BM, Castro Silva HF. Creación del valor en la cadena de abastecimiento del sector de salud en Colombia. Cuadernos de Administración. 2009;**22**(39):235-256

[4] Más-López CJ. La Contabilidad de Gestión y la formación de la cadena de valor en el sector de la salud: el costo de las enfermedades. Revista COFIN Habana. 2011;**5**(1):1-10

[5] Gálvez González A, García Fariñas A, Portuondo Sánchez C, Lara Bastanzuri C, Herrera M. Revista Cubana de Salud Pública. [Online]; [cited 2014 02 18]. 2012. Available from: http://scielo.sld.cu/scielo.php?script=sci_arttext&pid=S0864-34662012000200008&lng=es

[6] Más-López CJ. Libro electrónico: Investigaciones doctorales en las ciencias contables y administrativas. Procedimiento para calcular los costos de los tratamientos de la cirrosis hepática en el Instituto de Gastroenterología, considerando su cadena de valor extendida hacia los agentes sociales. Coordinadores: Jerónimo Ricárdez Jiménez y Francisco Borrás Atiénzar. ISBN: 978-607-9248-90-1. Universidad Veracruzana. Facultad de Contaduría y Administración. Veracruz, México; 2014

[7] Chapko M, Liu CF, Perkins M, Li YF, Fortney J, Maciejewski M. Equivalence of two healthcare costing methods: Bottom-up and top-down. Health Economy. 2009;**18**(10):1188-1201

[8] Espín Andrade AM. Factores de riesgo de carga en cuidadores informales de adultos mayores con demencia. Revista Cubana de Salud Pública. 2012;**38**(3):493-402

[9] Clabaugh G, Ward M. Cost-of-Illness studies in the United States: A systematic review of methodologies used for direct cost. Value Health. 2008;**11**(1):13-21

[10] Barrera Ortiz L, Sánchez Herrera B, Carrillo González GM. La carga del cuidado en cuidadores de niños con enfermedad crónica. Revista Cubana de Enfermería. 2013;**29**(1):39-47

[11] Liu JL, Maniadakis N, Gray A, Rayner M. The Economic Burden of Coronary Heart Disease in the UK. Heart. 2002;**17**(3):597-603

[12] Oliva J, Lobo L-BJ, Duque OR. Costes no sanitarios ocasionados por las enfermedades isquémicas del corazón en España. Cuadernos Económicos ICE. 2004;**67**(1):263-298

[13] Fernández-de-Bobadilla J, López-de-Sá E. Carga económica y social de la enfermedad coronaria. Revista española de cardiología suplementos. 2013;**13**(1):42-47

[14] Drummond M, Obrien B, Stoddart G, Torrance G. Métodos para la Evaluación Económica de los Programas de Asistencia. Sanitaria Madrid: Díaz de Santos; 2001

[15] Alfonso G. Marketing de servicios: Reinterpretando la cadena de valor. Palermo Business Review. 2008;**8**(2):56-69

[16] FAO. Designing and Implementing Livestock Value Chain Studies Guidelines. Roma: Food and Agriculture Organization of the United Nations (FAO); 2012

[17] King Núñez KI. gestiopolis.com. [Online]. 2012 [cited 2020 25]. Available from: https://www.gestiopolis.com/valor-compartido-teoria-michael-poter/

[18] Más López CJ. Revista Confin Habana Vol 8 No. 4. [Online]; [cited 2014 01 23]. 2013. Available from: http://cofinhabana.fcf.uh.cu/

[19] Aguayo Joza MJ. Procedimiento para calcular los costos del cáncer cervicouterino en Solca, Manabí. Ecuador. La Habana: Facultad de Contabilidad y Finanzas. Universidad de La Habana; 2020

[20] Gálvez González AM, Graber, Le Galès. Innovación y cuidados del cáncer en Cuba desde la evaluación socioeconómica y la etnocontabilidad. Información para directivos de la Salud. Sep-Dic; 2020;**32**(842):1-22

[21] Fernández García A, Triana Casado I, Villar VR. Costos directos del glaucoma primario del ángulo abierto. Revista Cubana de Salud Pública. 2006;**30**(1):51-66

[22] Fernández García A. Sielo. [Online]; [cited 2014 01 18]. 2011. Available from: http://scielo.sld.cu/>

[23] Way J. eHow. [Online]; [cited 2014 02 26]. 2014. Available from: http://www.ehow.com/info_8658888_activitybased-costing-method-accounting.html

[24] Harrington JH. Mejoramiento de los procesos de la empresa. Bogotá: McGraw-Hill; 1992

[25] Amat O, Soldevilla P. Contabilidad y Gestión de Costes. España: Editora Gestión; 2002

[26] Horngren TC, Datar MS, Rajan VM. Contabilidad de Costos. Un enfoque gerencial. Naucalpan de Juárez, México: Pearson Educación de México S.A de C.V (Decimocuarta edición); 2012

[27] Castelló TE. Los nuevos desafíos de la contabilidad de gestión. Boletín AECA No. 25. 1991. Available from: http://www.observatorio-iberoamericano.org/paises/Spain/Art%C3%ADculos%20diversos%20sobre%20Contabilidad%20de%20Gesti%C3%B3n/Nuevos%20de

[28] Baujín Pérez P. Evolución histórica de la contabilidad de gestión. 2005. Available from: https://www.gestiopolis.com/evolucion-historica-de-la-contabilidad-de-gestion

[29] Emblemsvag J. Emblemsvag Blog. [Online]; [cited 2014 02 26]. 2010. Available from: http://www.emblemsvag.com/abc.htm

[30] Porter ME. Ventaja Competitiva. Creación y Seguimiento de un Desempeño Superior. México D. F: Continental s.a; 1985

[31] Calderon JES, Campos AS. Eficacia de las pruebas diagnósticas del Cáncer Cervicouterino y Virus del Papiloma Humano. Journal of Negative and No Positive Results. 2019;**4**(5):551-566

[32] Ministerio de Salud Pública. Tarifario de prestaciones para el sistema nacional de salud. Acuerdo Ministerial 4928. Registro Oficial Edición Especial 235. Quito. Ecuador: Ministerio de Salud Pública.; 2014

[33] Capasso. El Costeo Objetivo. Buenos Aires. Argentina; 2015

[34] INEC. Encuesta Nacional de Ingresos y Gastos de Hogares Urbanos y Rurales. [Online]. Quito. Ecuador: Instituto Nacional de Estadísticas y Censos; 2012 [cited 2020, 25]. Available from: https://www.ecuadorencifras.gob.ec/documentos/webnec/Estadisticas_Sociales/Encuestas_Nac_Ingresos_Gastos_Hogares_Urb_Rur_ENIGHU/ENIGHU-2011-2012/Metodologia_ENIGHUR_2011-2012_rev.pdf

[35] Planifica Ecuador. Secretaria Técnica Planifica Ecuador. [Online]. 2019. Available from: www.planificacion.gob.es

Chapter 4

Cytologic Monitoring, Management of Cervical Cancer, and Control of Human Papillomavirus

Zakariyya Muhammad Bello, Sharafudeen Dahiru Abubakar, Imam Malik Kabir and Lukman Yusuf

Abstract

Cervical cancer is the second most common cause of cancer-related death among women that is caused by Human Papillomavirus, a double-stranded virus that leads to cellular alterations in the cervical squamocolumnar junction. Most HPV infections are cleared by the host immune system, while very low cases progress to invasive carcinoma due to persistent infection and other contributory risk factors. Several screening techniques have been devised over the years to detect Human Papillomavirus at an early stage, the most common being the Pap smear test, which is capable of detecting benign cellular changes and also squamous intraepithelial neoplasias. Other important techniques involve visual inspection with acetic acid (VIA), colposcopy, and HPV DNA testing. In addition, recent advances have led to the development of new techniques such as biosensor and bioreceptor technology and loop-mediated isothermal amplification (LAMP). Several methods have been in place to prevent the increased incidence of cervical cancer. Among these is the development of Prophylactic HPV vaccines, which elicit a humoral immune response against about 15 HPV genotypes but have the limitation of not curing an established cancer. Several trials are underway on developing a therapeutic vaccine that will be effective in curing cervical cancer.

Keywords: cervical cancer screening, cervical cancer management, HPV vaccine, HPV prevention, cervical cancer control

1. Introduction

Cervical cancer is the second-leading cause of global gynecological cancer-related deaths in women [1]. Human papillomavirus (HPV), a double-stranded DNA tumor virus, is the major cause of cervical cancer. Even though a strong immune system can normally fight off HPV infections, chronic infections with high-risk (HR) HPVs lead to cervical cancer [2]. However, in recent years, cancer patient assessment methods have changed from actual decision-making, based on the clinic-pathological characteristics of the patient, to biomarker-driven treatment plans, focusing on genetics and specific targeted medicines. Furthermore, the molecular alterations that occur during the development of cervical carcinogenesis have been examined using high-throughput technologies and gene expression profiling based on microarrays. The found genes with abnormal expression may aid in the diagnosis of cancer, the subtyping of cancer, and the design of chemotherapy [3, 4]. Also worthy of mentioning is the Papanicolaou (Pap) test that has been the primary option for gynecological screening for almost 60 years due to its ease of use, low cost, and lack of major side effects, which has likely contributed to its success in recent years in lowering overall incidence and mortality in the world [5]. Despite this, recent screening studies from several nations have showed the advantages of HPV testing over the Pap test for detecting cervical cancer, as HPV-based screening was 70% more efficient in reducing the incidence of invasive cervical carcinomas than cytology-based screening [6]. This study's goal is to highlight the importance of cytologic surveillance, cervical cancer treatment, and HPV prevention.

2. Current cervical cancer screening initiatives

HPV viral gene integration in the host genome promotes the expression of E6 and E7, with subsequent deadly genetic changes leading to neoplastic transformation. HPV-infected cells can advance from normal to preinvasive to invasive cancer in about 10 years or more [7]. However, this lengthy timeframe allows for the detection of early preinvasive neoplastic lesions and the prevention of cancer development through screening. Cervical cancer screening can be done in three ways, namely, VIA, Pap smear, and HPV DNA testing.

2.1 Pap test

George Papanicolaou established the Pap smear test in the early 1940s. A qualified cytotechnologist or pathologist will collect a liquid biopsy from the squamocolumnar junction and smear it on a glass slide for microscope examination. With a sensitivity of 70–80%, it is the earliest screening technique that became widely used in the 1960s [8]. The adequacy of the specimen is absolutely essential for the accuracy of the Pap test [9]. The cellular changes are reported in accordance with the "The Bethesda System for Reporting Cervical Cytology," which establishes consistent and reproducible criteria for detecting preinvasive and invasive cancer [10]. The most significant benefit of a traditional Pap smear technique is its cheapness and affordability [11]. Although the Pap test is successful in cities, it has failed in rural areas because it is an extremely competent personnel-intensive scheme. Key drawbacks include the low sensitivity to detect early preinvasive lesions, the complex logistical and care network necessary for executing quality control, and the succeeding relevant medical management (like colposcopy, histology, and endocervical curettage) of women who screen positive [12]. As a result, there is an urgent need to develop a reliable, highly sensitive, and cost-effective cervical cancer screening technique.

2.2 Visual inspection with acetic acid

Visual examination of the cervix while using 3% acetic acid offers an alternate, economically advantageous screening method [7]. The cervical dysplastic regions are highlighted by the application of acetic acid, which causes instantaneous color changes that are evident to the unaided eye. Any alteration in hue is considered a sign of cervical cancer that has not yet spread. Since the 1990s, visual inspection with acetic acid (VIA) has been employed, particularly in rural and remote areas. It is a straightforward, user-friendly method. The VIA technique has the distinct advantage that care providers can fulfill their duties without the need for sophisticated infrastructure or equipment [13]. According to the findings of Arbyn et al., VIA has a specificity of 81–89% as well as a sensitivity of 73–85% for identifying high-grade cervical preinvasive lesions [14]. Nevertheless, the VIA technique has limitations such as provider dependence and subjectivity, as well as lower sensitivity for women over the age of 40. This necessitates immediate action to develop an alternative approach with greater sensitivity, specificity, and noninvasiveness.

2.3 HPV DNA testing

The only circulating tumor DNA tests that have received clinical approval to date are quantitative PCR-based tests; however, other studies have shown that digital PCR and sequencing are preferred due to their enhanced capacity to identify uncommon variations. By finding variations without knowing their precise sequence, sequencing-based approaches dramatically boost flexibility. Due to the high expense and complexity of NGS, especially those approaches used for low-abundance mutations, sequencing studies must frequently concentrate on narrower regions of the genome where mutations are likely to occur [15]. Despite this, targeted assays have no sensitivity to mutations that they are not targeted to study; NGS approaches have a distinct benefit in that they discover variants with little to no prior information of the mutation's existence or position. This benefit is less pronounced when taking into account a number of prospective uses for ctDNA, such as companion diagnostics, where the pertinent mutations and related cautions are well-known and scarce [16]. In these circumstances, focused assays may outperform sequencing, especially if they can be carried out quickly, easily, and affordably. This is corroborated by the fact that digital PCR (dPCR), despite being virtually exclusively utilized for singleplex tests, is currently quite popular in preclinical research of ctDNA [17]. However, The Cobas 4800 HPV/DNA automated PCR equipment was effectively used in previous research from Sri Lanka to show that HPV-DNA testing can be used as a primary screening tool in low-resource settings [18]. Rapid molecular point-of-care assays for identifying HPV DNA have been developed recently [19]. While the HPV-DNA test is highly sensitive, it is less specific. Thus, it may be able to identify clinically inconsequential infections in women who are at risk of developing cervical cancer. Therefore, in order for these procedures to be truly effective in a diagnostic set, they ought not to be time-consuming and expensive. Also, they need to be highly specific.

2.4 Biosensor and aptamer technology

The most crucial aspect of a biosensor is likely selectivity. The capacity of a bioreceptor to identify a particular analyte in a sample that contains various admixtures and impurities is known as selectivity. The relationship between an antigen and an antibody provides the best illustration of selectivity. Traditionally, antibodies function as bioreceptors and are immobilized on the transducer's surface. The antigen-containing solution is then exposed to the transducer, where antibodies only interact with the antigens. The solution is typically a buffer including salts. Selectivity is the primary factor to be taken into account when selecting bioreceptors for a biosensor [20]. Furthermore, reproducibility, or the biosensor's capacity to produce the same results under equal experimental conditions, is another quality of a successful biosensor. The transducer and electronics in a biosensor are precise and accurate, which defines reproducibility. When a sample is tested more than once, accuracy refers to the sensor's capability to offer a mean value that is close to the true value, while precision refers to the sensor's ability to produce identical findings every time. The inference made on a biosensor's response is highly reliable and robust when the signals are reproducible. A biosensor's sensitivity is one of its key characteristics. Besides this, a biosensor's limit of detection (LOD), or sensitivity, is determined by the smallest amount of analyte that it can detect. Additionally, the stability of a biosensing system determines how susceptible it is to environmental disturbances both inside and outside of it. A biosensor under measurement may experience a drift in its output signals as a result of these disruptions. This could skew the concentration being measured and compromise the biosensor's precision and accuracy. In applications where a biosensor needs lengthy incubation periods or ongoing monitoring, stability is the most important component. The reaction of electronics and transducers may be temperature-sensitive, which could affect a biosensor's stability. To achieve a steady response from the sensor, proper tuning of the electronics is necessary as shown in **Figure 1**. Likewise, linearity is the property that demonstrates the precision of the measured response to a straight line for a measurement set with various analyte concentrations. It is mathematically represented as $y = mc$, where c is the analyte concentration, y is the output signal, and m is the sensitivity of the biosensor. The

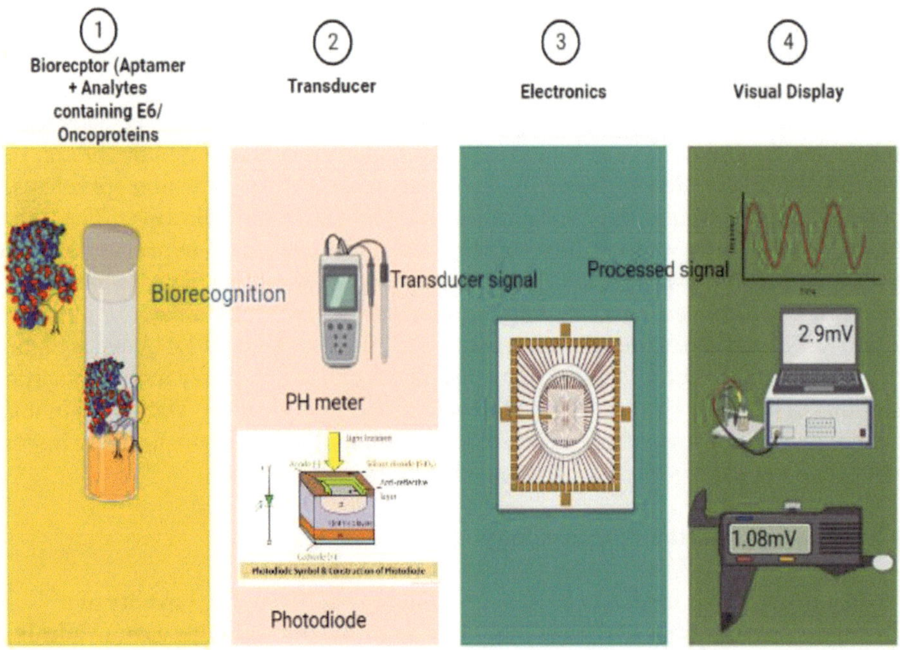

Figure 1.
An illustration of a biosensor in diagrammatic form. 1. The analyte E6/7 oncoproteins are particularly recognized by the aptamer molecule. Upon the engagement of the bioreceptor with the analyte, the process of bio-recognition occurs, during which a signal is produced (in the form of light or pH). 2. The transducer converts the bio-recognition event into a measurable signal. 3. The transduced signal is processed by the electronics and made ready for display. It is made up of intricate electrical circuitry that carries out signal conditioning tasks like signal amplification as well as conversion from analog to digital form. 4. The display produces user-friendly numerical results.

resolution of the biosensor and the range of analyte concentrations under test can both affect the biosensor's linearity. The smallest change in an analyte's concentration necessary to cause a change in the biosensor's response is known as the resolution of the biosensor. A strong resolution may be necessary depending on the application since biosensor applications call for the detection of analyte concentrations over a large operating range [20]. Generally, there are different ways that biosensors can be used to enhance the quality of life. This area includes their application for a variety of purposes, including environmental monitoring, disease detection, food safety, and drug development. The detection of biomolecules that are either disease indicators or medication targets is one of the main uses for biosensors. For instance, clinical tools for the detection of protein cancer biomarkers can be developed using electrochemical biosensing techniques [21]. Yet these methods have the ability to use aptamers to detect these biomolecules [22]. Aptamers are easily synthesized and available for purchase once they have been created. Aptamers not only have a high affinity and specificity for their target while undergoing a conformational change, but they can also maintain the majority of their functionality even after going through several regeneration steps [23]. Moreover, they are easily adaptable to other functional groups, allowing for a wider range of applications [24]. Electrochemical biosensors have always been a hot topic in research because of their ease of use, low cost, high sensitivity, quick turnaround, and resilient nature. They also only need basic apparatus. There are numerous studies in the literature on impedimetric aptasensors that take advantage of the aptamers' conformational change capabilities as well as other elements that alter the system's impedance [25].

2.5 Loop-mediated isothermal amplification

Digital PCR and NGS have often been preferred for ctDNA studies. However, LAMP could be used to replace these approaches because it has proven to be inexpensive, efficient, and highly specific, in addition to having reasonable sensitivity. Meanwhile, the method begins with cell-free DNA extraction and analysis as described in earlier studies [26]. As the HPV ctDNA can be amplified without the DNA extraction stage, therefore this step can be avoided. Even though PCR was employed to amplify the HPV ctDNA genes disclosed in the listed papers, LAMP can be used as its substitute. Milan et al. recommended the use of an electrochemical LAMP-based test to identify HPV16/18 infection in cervical samples. The LAMP reaction was performed in the aforementioned study using a premixed mixture of WarmStart LAMP 2 Master Mix, DIG-dUTP, 100 ng of DNA template, and LAMP primers. They performed the process at 66°C for 40 min, following a polymerase inactivation at 80°C for 5 min. Subsequently, Agarose gel electrophoresis was used to detect the LAMP reaction on 1.5% agarose gel stained with GelRed nucleic acid. Nevertheless, based on the identification of the amplicons, there are numerous LAMP models available. Anton et al., on the other hand, preferred to combine electrochemical measurements with a geomagnetic technique, using streptavidin magnetic beads to assess DIG-labeled LAMP amplicons in a working electrode [27]. In yet another work by Mudhigeti et al. the LAMP mixture with sample-containing tubes was placed in a water bath that had been preheated to 63°C for 60 minutes [28]. Following a brief exposure to blue light, 1 l of SYBR Green I was added to each tube, gently mixed, and checked for bright green fluorescence. Bright green fluorescence denotes the presence of the target (HPV) or successful amplification, while no fluorescence denotes the target's absence. Likewise, Yu et al. used digital LAMP assays on a self-digitization

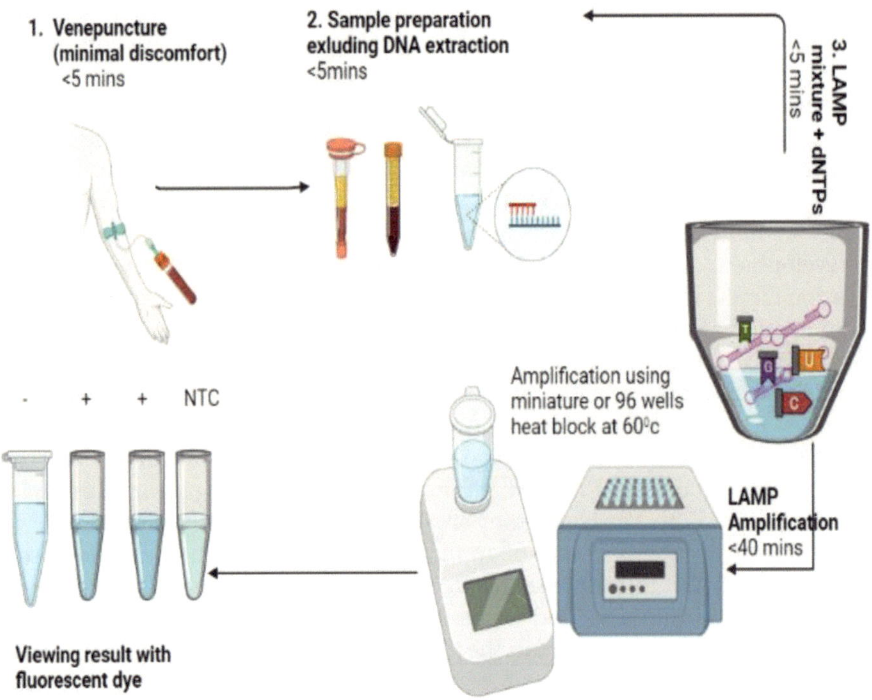

Figure 2.
Employing LAMP in the diagnosis of HPV ctDNA Summary of the procedure. About 5mls of blood will be collected. 2. Sample will be separated, it can either be extracted or amplified directly. 3. LAMP mixture will be added to an Eppendorf tube containing the sample. 4. At a single temperature of about 600c the HPV ctDNA will be amplified 5. The positive sample can be viewed with the naked eye either through turbidity of color intensity using fluorescent dye.

chip to detect 14 high-risk human papillomaviruses [29]. All of these studies used LAMP to detect HPV DNA in the cervical sample, but so far, no report has yet been published on the detection of HPV ctDNA using LAMP. The summary of this procedure is depicted in **Figure 2**.

3. Cervical cancer control

The global strategy developed by WHO for cervical cancer elimination has proposed three essential ways to fight HPV; 90% of girls fully vaccinated with the HPV vaccine by the age of 15 years, high-performance cervical screening of 70% of women at 35 and 45 years of age, and 90% treatment of infected women with confirmed cervical cancer. These targets must be met by 2030 for countries to be on the path toward cervical cancer elimination [30]. To achieve this goal, WHO with its partners is developing a global strategy toward the elimination of cervical cancer. Given the substantial global burden of cervical cancer, the increasing inequalities, and opportunities for effective and cost-effective primary and secondary prevention, the WHO Director-General made a global call in May 2018 for action toward eliminating cervical cancer as a public health problem [31]. A comprehensive national or sub-national surveillance system for elimination would encompass long-term surveillance of both processes and outcomes across the three core activities of vaccination, screening, and treatment as outlined in the WHO Global Strategy toward eliminating cervical cancer as a public health problem [32].

3.1 HPV vaccine

Large international randomized control clinical trials have proved that HPV vaccines are safe and highly effective against vaccine-type infection and cervical precancerous lesions in women (with vaccine efficacy ≥93%). These vaccines target high-risk HPV types that cause about 70% (bivalent and quadrivalent vaccines: HPV types 16 and 18) and 90% (9-valent vaccine: HPV types 16, 18, 31, 33, 45, 52, and 58) of cervical cancers [31]. Large-scale international randomized control clinical trials have demonstrated the safety and great efficacy of HPV vaccinations in preventing vaccine-type infections and cervical precancerous lesions in females (vaccine efficacy of 93%). These vaccines target high-risk HPV types that account for 70% (HPV types 16 and 18 in the bivalent and quadrivalent vaccines) and 90% (HPV types 16, 18, 31, 33, 45, 52, and 58 in the 9-valent vaccine) of cervical malignancies, respectively [31]. The currently available HPV vaccines were created using the virus-like particles (VLPs) of the primary papillomavirus capsid protein L1, which are essentially empty viral shells made up of one or more different polymeric shells or capsid proteins [33]. All three HPV vaccines were developed based on L1 VLP [33]. VLPs are not infectious or carcinogenic because they lack a viral genome that is capable of eliciting a humoral immune response with significant and persistent neutralizing antibodies [33].

Early genes are thus targeted during the viral life cycle and aid in regulating the emergence of HPV-related premalignant and malignant abrasions. Because E6 and E7 proteins are continually produced and connected to the malignant development of HPV-linked malignancies, they provide two promising targets for therapeutic HPV vaccines. Other proteins E1 (viral helicase) and E2 are useful for focusing on early viral abrasions, and these proteins are expressed at a faster rate than E6 and E7 before viral genome incorporation at early stages [34].

The three HPV prophylactic vaccines currently available are, respectively, Gardasil®4, a quadrivalent vaccine available in 2006 [35]; Cervarix™, a bivalent vaccine available in 2007 [36]; and Gardasil®9, a nonavalent vaccine available in 2014 [37]. Both the quadrivalent and bivalent vaccines show varying degrees of protection against oncogenic HPV types not included in the vaccines [38]. Data from clinical trials showed that these three vaccines all achieved good preventive effects on people infected by HPV from different regions, of different races, and in different age groups. Moreover, the majority of trial data for several vaccines provided vaccine titers data against advanced cervical cancer precursors (CIN 2, CIN 3, and adenocarcinoma *in situ*) [33].

To eliminate tumors or lesions, the vaccine unleashes T-cell immunity by directly targeting HPV antigens exposed around infected and malignant cells [34]. These proteins can be good targets for therapeutic vaccines since vaccines can target cytotoxic T lymphocytes (CTLs) and cancer-specific T cell type 1 that can destroy cancer and infected cells [34].

3.2 Health education

The World Health Organization (WHO), as well as numerous studies and clinical registries on cancer survival, claims that developed nations with well-managed cervical cancer programs have seen a significant decline in cervical cancer incidence and mortality, but developing nations with low vaccination rates and weak cervical cancer screening programs have not [30]. For the past few decades, mortality and incidence rates have decreased in the majority of the world's regions. The decreases are attributed to elements that are associated with either rising socioeconomic averages or a declining risk of persistent infection with high-risk HPV as a result of advances in genital cleanliness, decreased parity, and a declining prevalence of sexually transmitted diseases [39]. Even though there are currently efforts to expand HPV vaccination as a means to prevent cervical cancer, in most African countries, it is still limited to research settings or poorly organized and with a slow rollout. In some countries, it is unavailable due to inadequate infrastructure, finances, and availability of healthcare workers. There are few countries that offer HPV vaccination through subsidized national immunization programs [40].

Many studies have suggested that low levels of public health education and knowledge of the disease, inadequate and inaccessibility of cervical cancer screening services, cultural beliefs, and perceived susceptibility contribute to the low cervical cancer screening rates [41, 42]. Lack of knowledge and awareness has been identified as one of the main reasons associated with low cervical cancer screening. Nonadherence to cervical cancer screening has been associated with a knowledge deficit [40]. Women living in rural settlements are mostly of low socioeconomic status, and this has been shown to be associated with a higher risk of cervical cancer, poor health knowledge, and poor access to health services [43].

Interventions utilizing peer health educators and culturally tailored methods were the most effective in improving screening uptake. Innovative approaches such as self-collected HPV testing can also be employed as they demonstrate the potential to influence changes in the uptake of screening [40]. Olubodun and coworkers reported that there is a need for increased cervical cancer awareness and promotion campaigns. Women's partners should also be targeted for health education. Improving access to cervical cancer prevention services is also crucial among this underserved population. Health education interventions increased knowledge and awareness of cervical cancer and boosted cancer screening. Therefore, a comprehensive approach to cervical cancer prevention and control should therefore include health education interventions [43].

4. Conclusion

Several efforts have been made to curtail the surge of cervical cancer incidence worldwide including early screening, vaccination, health education, HPV DNA testing, phylogenetic studies, and new molecular diagnostic techniques such as loop-mediated isothermal amplification and DNA-Aptamer-based biosensors. However, most of the new techniques are impracticable in resource-limited settings. Due to this, several efforts have been placed including health education and development of therapeutic HPV vaccines with ongoing clinical trials that lasted almost 20 years to date. It is expected that these vaccines will be able to cure or cause the regression of established cervical cancer, in addition to preventing recurrence. Therefore, hands on deck are needed to prevent the increased incidence of cervical cancer.

Conflict of interest

The authors declare no conflict of interest.

Acronyms and abbreviations

VIA	visual inspection with acetic acid
LAMP	loop-mediated isothermal amplification
HPV	human papillomavirus
Pap	papanicolaou test
PCR	polymerase chain reaction
NGS	next-generation sequencing
LOD	limit of detection
VLPs	virus-like particles
CIN	cervical cancer intraepithelial neoplasia

Author details

Zakariyya Muhammad Bello[1,2*], Sharafudeen Dahiru Abubakar[1,3], Imam Malik Kabir[2,4] and Lukman Yusuf[5]

1 Department of Medical Laboratory Science, College of Medical Sciences, Ahmadu Bello University, Zaria, Nigeria

2 Experimental Pathology Laboratory, Federal University of São João del-Rei (UFSJ), Divinópolis, Minas Gerais, Brazil

3 Research Institute for Biomedical Science, Tokyo University of Science, Japan

4 Department of Medical Laboratory Science, Bayero University, Kano, Nigeria

5 Kebbi State College of Health Sciences and Technology, Jega, Kebbi State, Nigeria

*Address all correspondence to: zakariyyab10@gmail.com; bzmuhammad@abu.edu.ng

References

[1] de Martel C, Plummer M, Vignat J, Franceschi S. Worldwide burden of cancer attributable to HPV by site, country and HPV type. International Journal of Cancer. 2017;**141**(4):664-670. DOI: 10.1002/ijc.30716

[2] Torre LA, Bray F, Siegel RL, Ferlay J, Lortet-Tieulent J, Jemal A. Global cancer statistics, 2012. CA: A Cancer Journal for Clinicians. 2015;**65**(2):87-108. DOI: 10.3322/caac.21262

[3] Chen Y, Miller C, Mosher R, Zhao X, Deeds J, Morrissey M, et al. Identification of cervical cancer markers by cDNA and tissue microarrays. Cancer Research. 2003;**63**(8):1927-1935

[4] Rajkumar T, Sabitha K, Vijayalakshmi N, Shirley S, Bose MV, Gopal G, et al. Identification and validation of genes involved in cervical tumorigenesis. BMC Cancer. 2011;**11**:80. DOI: 10.1186/1471-2407-11-80

[5] Comparetto C, Borruto F. Genetic screening of cervical cancer. OBM Genetics. 2021;**5**(3):1-37

[6] Suh DH, Kim M, Kim HJ, Lee KH, Kim JW. Major clinical research advances in gynecologic cancer in 2015. Journal of Gynecologic Oncology. 2016;**27**(6):e53. DOI: 10.3802/jgo.2016.27.e53

[7] Narasimhamurthy M, Kafle SU. Cervical cancer in Nepal: Current screening strategies and challenges. Frontiers in Public Health. 2022;**10**:980899. DOI: 10.3389/fpubh.2022.980899

[8] Soost HJ, Lange HJ, Lehmacher W, Ruffing-Kullmann B. The validation of cervical cytology. Sensitivity, specificity and predictive values. Acta Cytologica. 1991;**35**(1):8-14

[9] Martin-Hirsch P, Lilford R, Jarvis G, Kitchener HC. Efficacy of cervical-smear collection devices: A systematic review and meta-analysis. Lancet. 1999;**354**(9192):1763-1770. DOI: 10.1016/s0140-6736(99)02353-3

[10] Nayar R, Wilbur DC. The Bethesda System for Reporting Cervical Cytology: Definitions, Criteria, and Explanatory Notes. 3rd ed. Cham: Springer; 2015. DOI: 10.1007/978-3-319-11,074-5

[11] Mitteldorf CAT. Cervical cancer screening: From pap smear to future strategies. Jornal Brasileiro de Patologia e Medicina Laboratorial. 2016;**52**:238-245

[12] Basu P, Mittal S, Bhadra VD, Chami KY. Secondary prevention of cervical cancer. Best Practice & Research. Clinical Obstetrics & Gynaecology. 2018;**47**:73-85. DOI: 10.1016/j.bpobgyn.2017.08.012

[13] Sankaranarayanan R, Rajkumar R, Esmy PO, Fayette JM, Shanthakumary S, Frappart L, et al. Effectiveness, safety and acceptability of 'see and treat' with cryotherapy by nurses in a cervical screening study in India. British Journal of Cancer. 2007;**96**(5):738-743. DOI: 10.1038/sj.bjc.6603633

[14] Arbyn M, Sankaranarayanan R, Muwonge R, Keita N, Dolo A, Mbalawa CG, et al. Pooled analysis of the accuracy of five cervical cancer screening tests assessed in eleven studies in Africa and India. International Journal of Cancer. 2008;**123**(1):153-160. DOI: 10.1002/ijc.23489

[15] Rodda AE, Parker BJ, Spencer A, Corrie SR. Extending circulating tumor DNA analysis to ultralow abundance mutations: Techniques and challenges. ACS Sensors. 2018;**3**(3):540-560. DOI: 10.1021/acssensors.7b00953

[16] Lee H, Choi M, Lim J, Jo M, Han JY, Kim TM, et al. Magnetic nanowire networks for dual-isolation and detection of tumor-associated circulating biomarkers. Theranostics. 2018;**8**(2):505-517. DOI: 10.7150/thno.21967

[17] Volik S, Alcaide M, Morin RD, Collins C. Cell-free DNA (cfDNA): Clinical significance and utility in cancer shaped by emerging technologies. Molecular Cancer Research. 2016;**14**(10):898-908. DOI: 10.1158/1541-7786.MCR-16-0044

[18] Perera KCM, Mapitigama N, Abeysena H. The feasibility of new HPV/DNA test as a primary cervical cancer screening method among 35- years- old ever-married women in Kalutara district; A cross-sectional study. BMC Public Health. 2021;**21**(1):131. DOI: 10.1186/s12889-021-10,190-4

[19] Einstein MH, Smith KM, Davis TE, Schmeler KM, Ferris DG, Savage AH, et al. Clinical evaluation of the cartridge-based GeneXpert human papillomavirus assay in women referred for colposcopy. Journal of Clinical Microbiology. 2014;**52**(6):2089-2095. DOI: 10.1128/JCM.00176-14

[20] Bhalla N, Jolly P, Formisano N, Estrela P. Biosensor Technologies for Detection of Biomolecules. Portland Press; 31 Jul 2016

[21] Jolly P, Formisano N, Tkac J, Kasak P, Frost C, Estrela P. Label-free impedimetric Aptasensor with antifouling surface chemistry: A prostate specific antigen case study. Sensors and Actuators B: Chemical. 2015;**209**:306-312. DOI: 10.1016/j.snb.2014.11.083

[22] Buglak AA, Samokhvalov AV, Zherdev AV, Dzantiev BB. Methods and applications of In silico aptamer design and Modeling. International Journal of Molecular Sciences. 2020;**21**(22):8420. DOI: 10.3390/ijms21228420

[23] Sun S, Liu H, Hu Y, Wang Y, Zhao M, Yuan Y, et al. Selection and identification of a novel ssDNA aptamer targeting human skeletal muscle. Bioactive Materials. 2022;**20**:166-178. DOI: 10.1016/j.bioactmat.2022.05.016

[24] Sheng L, Ren J, Miao Y, Wang J, Wang E. PVP-coated graphene oxide for selective determination of ochratoxin a via quenching fluorescence of free aptamer. Biosensors & Bioelectronics. 2011;**26**(8):3494-3499. DOI: 10.1016/j.bios.2011.01.032

[25] Kumar VS, Kummari S, Catanante G, Gobi KV, Marty JL, Goud KY. A label-free impedimetric immunosensor for zearalenone based on CS-CNT-Pd nanocomposite modified screen-printed disposable electrodes. Sensors and Actuators B: Chemical. 2023;**377**:133077

[26] Sastre-Garau X, Diop M, Martin F, Dolivet G, Marchal F, Charra-Brunaud C, et al. A NGS-based blood test for the diagnosis of invasive HPV-associated carcinomas with extensive viral genomic characterization. Clinical Cancer Research. 2021;**27**(19):5307-5316. DOI: 10.1158/1078-0432.CCR-21-0293

[27] Anton M, Moranova L, Hrstka R, Bartosik M. Application of an electrochemical LAMP-based assay for screening of HPV16/HPV18 infection in cervical samples. Analytical Methods. 2020;**12**:822-829

[28] Mudhigeti N, Kalawat U, Hulikal N, Kante M. Evaluation of loop-mediated isothermal amplification assay for detection and typing of human papilloma virus 16 and 18 from endocervical samples. Indian Journal of Medical Microbiology. 2019;**37**(2):241-247. DOI: 10.4103/ijmm.IJMM_19_58

[29] Yu Z, Lyu W, Yu M, Wang Q, Qu H, Ismagilov RF, et al. Self-partitioning SlipChip for slip-induced droplet formation and human papillomavirus viral load quantification with digital LAMP. Biosensors & Bioelectronics. 2020;**155**:112107. DOI: 10.1016/j.bios.2020.112107

[30] World Health Organization. Global Strategy to Accelerate the Elimination of Cervical Cancer as a Public Health Problem. World Health Organization; 31 Dec 2020. Available from: https://apps.who.int/iris/handle/10665/336583

[31] Brisson M, Kim JJ, Canfell K, Drolet M, Gingras G, Burger EA, et al. Impact of HPV vaccination and cervical screening on cervical cancer elimination: A comparative modelling analysis in 78 low-income and lower-middle-income countries. Lancet. 2020;**395**(10224):575-590. DOI: 10.1016/S0140-6736(20)30068-4

[32] Brotherton JML, Wheeler C, Clifford GM, Elfström M, Saville M, Kaldor J, et al. Surveillance systems for monitoring cervical cancer elimination efforts: Focus on HPV infection, cervical dysplasia, cervical screening and treatment. Preventive Medicine. 2021;**144**:106293. DOI: 10.1016/j.ypmed.2020.106293

[33] Mo Y, Ma J, Zhang H, Shen J, Chen J, Hong J, et al. Prophylactic and therapeutic HPV vaccines: Current scenario and perspectives. Frontiers in Cellular and Infection Microbiology. 2022;**12**:909223. DOI: 10.3389/fcimb.2022.909223

[34] Ayesha N, Aboulaghras S, Jahangeer M, Riasat A, Ramzan R, Fatima R, et al. Physiopathology and effectiveness of therapeutic vaccines against human papillomavirus. Environmental Science and Pollution Research International. 2021;**28**(35):47752-47772. DOI: 10.1007/s11356-021-15,441-w

[35] Hanna E, Bachmann G. HPV vaccination with Gardasil: A breakthrough in Women's health. Expert Opinion on Biological Therapy. 2006;**6**(11):1223-1227. DOI: 10.1517/14712598.6.11.1223

[36] Crosbie EJ, Kitchener HC. Cervarix–a bivalent L1 virus-like particle vaccine for prevention of human papillomavirus type 16- and 18- associated cervical cancer. Expert Opinion on Biological Therapy. 2007;**7**(3):391-396. DOI: 10.1517/14712598.7.3.391

[37] Printz C. FDA approves Gardasil 9 for more types of HPV. Cancer. 2015;**121**(8):1156-1157. DOI: 10.1002/cncr.29374

[38] Jit M, Chapman R, Hughes O, Choi YH. Comparing bivalent and quadrivalent human papillomavirus vaccines: Economic evaluation based on transmission model. British Medical Journal. 2011;**343**:d5775. DOI: 10.1136/bmj.d5775

[39] Sung H, Ferlay J, Siegel RL, Laversanne M, Soerjomataram I, Jemal A, et al. Global cancer statistics 2020: GLOBOCAN estimates of incidence and mortality worldwide for 36 cancers in 185 countries. CA: A Cancer Journal for Clinicians. 2021;**71**(3):209-249. DOI: 10.3322/caac.21660

[40] Makadzange EE, Peeters A, Joore MA, Kimman ML. The effectiveness of health education interventions on cervical cancer prevention in Africa: A systematic review. Preventive Medicine. 2022;**164**:107219. DOI: 10.1016/j.ypmed.2022.107219

[41] Binka C, Nyarko SH, Awusabo-Asare K, Doku DT. Barriers to the uptake of cervical cancer screening and treatment among rural

women in Ghana. BioMed Research International. 2019;**2019**:6320938. DOI: 10.1155/2019/6320938

[42] Ducray JF, Kell CM, Basdav J, Haffejee F. Cervical cancer knowledge and screening uptake by marginalized population of women in inner-city Durban, South Africa: Insights into the need for increased health literacy. Womens Health (Lond). 2021;**17**:17455065211047141. DOI: 10.1177/17455065211047141

[43] Olubodun T, Odukoya OO, Balogun MR. Knowledge, attitude and practice of cervical cancer prevention, among women residing in an urban slum in Lagos, South West, Nigeria. The Pan African Medical Journal. 2019;**32**:130. DOI: 10.11604/pamj.2019.32.130.14432